PLAB

PART 1 EMQ

POCKET BOOK 3

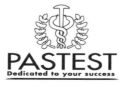

PASTEST
Dedicated to your success

PLAB
PART 1 EMQ
POCKET BOOK 3

John Buchanan

BSc(Hons), MFDS, RCPS(Glas), MRCP
Specialist Registrar
Oral Medicine
Eastman Dental Hospital
UCLH London

Andrea Hermann

MD, DFFP, MRCOG, MRCP
Specialist Registrar
Department of Obstetrics & Gynaecology
Princess Margaret Hospital
Swindon

Hank Schneider

Consultant General and Paediatric Surgeon
Department of Surgery
The James Paget Hospital
Great Yarmouth
Norfolk

Kithsiri A Withana

MBBS, FRCP, FRCPCH, DCH, DTCH
Consultant Paediatrician
Paediatric Department
Chase Farm Hospital
Middlesex

© 2002 PASTEST LTD
Egerton Court, Parkgate Estate,
Knutsford, Cheshire, WA16 8DX
Telephone: 01565 752000

First edition 2002
Reprinted 2003

A catalogue record for this book is available from the British Library.

ISBN: 1 901198 70 7

The information contained within this book was obtained by the author from reliable sources. However, while every effort has been made to ensure its accuracy, no responsibility for loss, damage or injury occasioned to any person acting or refraining from action as a result of information contained herein can be accepted by the publishers or authors.

Typeset by Breeze Limited, Manchester
Printed by Ashford Colour Press Ltd, Gosport, Hampshire

CONTENTS

INTRODUCTION

About this book

Congratulations on buying this book!

Unfortunately, not everyone can pass PLAB Part 1 first time. Amazingly, many candidates do not buy any books or go on any courses. Whilst using this book, or any book, cannot guarantee a pass at the next exam, it will certainly improve your chances.

The proportion of candidates that pass is fixed at each sitting. Therefore, you are in competition with everyone that sits the exam at the same time as you. If you help one of your friends with their revision, you may be helping them pass instead of you. Group learning is, of course, often of great benefit, but be careful that you are not helping others more than yourself. For your own sake, do not lend this book to anyone else until you have passed the exam…

This book is not a textbook. You will not find great detail and many topics could not be included in the space available. A small textbook or guide (such as the Oxford Handbook series) is recommended for revision. Subjects like paediatrics, obstetrics and psychiatry seem popular with the examiners. If you are weak in these areas, it might be worth obtaining small books dedicated to these specialties. Do not spend too much time or money on new, large textbooks. You will never read them.

This book is not, strictly speaking, a revision book. There are very few lists in the text. Again, this is partly due to the limited number of topics that could be covered. Also, there are some very good books of lists and differential diagnosis already in print. If you like lists and your memory can cope with them, then it may be worth buying one of these books.

If you are new to the exam, this book will introduce you to the type of question that you will be facing. For those of you who have already sat the new exam (since July 2000), the book provides another 200 practice questions. Many difficult questions are made easier by understanding the way in which an examiner might think. I hope to provide some insight into the way in which the questions and answers are designed. This is particularly important now that the General Medical Council (GMC) has changed the format of the exam.

Introduction

The new exam and why it was changed

The General Medical Council (GMC) frequently reviews the way in which it examines overseas doctors in the PLAB process. Ultimately the exam may be replaced by another form of assessment. In the meantime, the GMC is keen to make the exam fairer and open to independent scrutiny. The previous Part 1 (multiple choice, picture and clinical problem-solving questions) was not felt to be a fair test of knowledge and ability.

A number of books were available for the previous model of exam. If you have any of these books, do not throw them away. The topics that are covered are still those that the PLAB exam will test. Incidentally, there is no guarantee that the exam format will not change again in the future.

Multiple choice questions (MCQs) are particularly subject to criticism. The current exam consists of Extended Matching Questions (EMQs), closely modelled on the style of exams in the USA. According to the GMC, the level of knowledge required to pass the exam should be roughly the same as before. At the first sitting of the new exam (July 2000), it was felt to be harder than expected by many candidates.

The GMC states that the standard required is that of a first year Senior House Officer, i.e. someone with 12 to 18 months experience since qualification. Some questions in July 2000 were almost certainly harder than that and seemed to expect greater depth of knowledge. Do not let this discourage you. A hard exam is equally hard on everyone. An easy exam is more likely to let weaker candidates pass by luck alone.

Many candidates do not always answer all 200 questions, you will need to practice using the time wisely. There will always be a few questions that you struggle with, try to waste as little time as possible on these. Put down an educated guess and move on quickly to a question you feel more confident about. This will boost your morale and produce greater time efficiency.

Since July 2000 there have been no picture questions in the Part 1 exam. The GMC would not commit to whether picture questions will be reintroduced in the future.

Are EMQs harder than MCQs?

This is a difficult question to answer. MCQs are easy to set and mark. They test recall (often short term memory) and do not attempt to simulate clinical reality. A guess at multiple choice gives you a 50/50 chance of a correct answer. So does tossing a coin. An educated guess is often not much better due to the nature of the question. You either know it, or you don't.

EMQs are much harder to write. They test knowledge and deduction and often attempt to simulate clinical problem-solving. A random guess is unlikely to produce a correct answer when there may be as many as 14 possibilities. An educated guess is more likely to be right than wrong.

EMQs are probably a better test of knowledge and experience than MCQs. In clinical practice, if a 25-year-old man attends casualty with left-sided chest pain you do not think like this:

'Sudden unilateral chest pain in a 25-year-old man is commonly due to
pulmonary embolism – True
pneumothorax – True
dissecting thoracic aortic aneurysm – False'

Whereas you might think the following:

'The most likely cause of sudden left-sided chest pain in a 25-year-old
man is a pneumothorax'

EMQs also test the application of knowledge. In the July 2000 exam, most of the questions asked candidates to select the best investigation, rather than the most likely diagnosis. This is also relevant to clinical practice and harder to answer. When faced with the patient with chest pain, you will have a differential diagnosis and need to plan investigations to decide which diagnosis is correct. You may think the differential diagnosis is between pneumothorax, pulmonary embolism and oesophagitis. You must then decide whether a chest X-ray, arterial blood gases or an endoscopy is the investigation of choice. There may not be one single investigation that will establish the diagnosis in all circumstances, so you must pick the most discriminatory one. In this instance, a chest X-ray is probably the most useful test.

In answer to the question 'are EMQs harder than MCQs?', the answer is probably 'Yes'. However, they are a better and fairer test of clinical ability.

Doctors who pass this new exam will be those who have combined reading with hands-on experience. The previous Part 1 exam could, potentially, be passed by someone who had never seen a patient.

How to use this book

This book is designed as a complete mock PLAB Part 1 Examination. In the front section of this book there are 200 EMQs covering a wide selection of topics. The second section has answers to the questions with detailed, but not exhaustive, explanations to the answers. In the appendix, you will find a table of normal values for standard laboratory tests and a list of useful addresses.

Endeavour to use the practice exam **under strict examination conditions**: make sure you set aside a full three hours for the exam, preferably during the daytime when the real exam will take place. Make sure you are not disturbed in any way – unplug the telephone, do not have any background music on and make sure your partner or flatmate is out of the way.

Work systematically through the exam paper from the beginning. Previous candidates found that some questions were considerably harder than others. If a question is obviously difficult, miss it out and move on to the next one. If the whole topic is unfamiliar to you, move on to the next one. Two minutes are more efficiently spent answering two easy questions than puzzling over one hard question. When you reach the end of the paper, go back to the questions you missed out until you run out of time. Three hours is not a long time to answer 200 questions, you have slightly less than one minute per question.

When the three hours have finished, stop answering questions. Relax and treat yourself, you deserve it!

When you are refreshed, come back and finish any questions you did not answer during the time on a separate sheet of paper. If you completed all 200 questions, well done! If not, have a go at all the others – an educated guess is often the right answer. Then go through the answers and mark the questions you managed during the time and see how you did. Look at the other questions separately. Use the explanations to identify areas of strength and weakness to guide your revision. It is difficult to say what score you will need to pass the exam, as the pass mark will vary at each sitting, depending on the difficulty of the exam. I would expect that a score of at least 50–60% would be a bare minimum to pass. In January 2001, the pass rate was 60%.

Introduction

It is unlikely that you will remember many of the questions in this book for long. About a week before the real thing, it will be worth trying this practice exam again. In using this book, you are making sure that the exam is not the first time you have encountered this type of question. Hopefully, the next PLAB Part 1 Exam will be the last one you have to take.

Referring to our Revision Checklist at the back of this book will ensure that you cover the most popular examination themes.

Good Luck!

RECOMMENDED READING LIST

1. **Shorter Books which may be useful for Revision**

   Use **one** of these three:
   Lecture Notes on Clinical Medicine
   D Rubenstein and D Wayne, Blackwell Scientific Publications, 1997

   Oxford Handbook of Clinical Medicine
   R A Hope and J M Longmore, Oxford University Press, 1998

   Essential Medicine
   A E Read and J V Jones, Churchill Livingstone, 1998

   Both of these are also worth reading:
   Oxford Handbook of Clinical Specialities
   J A B Collier, J M Longmore and T J Hodgetts, Oxford University Press,
   4th edition 1995

   Essential Paediatrics
   D Hull and D I Johnston, Churchill Livingstone (also available as an
   International Student Edition)

2. **Books which are too long or detailed for revision but should be
   useful for reference**

   Acute Medicine
   D C Sprigings and J B Chambers, Blackwell Scientific Publications,
   2nd edition 1995.

   Medical Emergencies – Diagnosis and Management
   R Robinson and R B Stott, Butterworth Heinemann, 6th edition 1993

   Clinical Medicine
   P J Kumar and M L Clark, Balliere Tindall, 1998

   Textbook of Medicine
   R Souhami and J Moxham, Churchill Livingstone, 1997

   Lecture Notes on General Surgery
   H Ellis and R Calne, Blackwell Scientific Publications, 1998

Recommended Reading List

Handbook of General Surgery
P G Bevan and I A Donovan, Blackwell Scientific Publications, 1992

Concise System of Orthopaedics and Fractures
A G Apley and L Solomon, Butterworth Heinemann, 2nd edition 1994

Lecture Notes on Orthopaedics and Fractures
T Duckworth, Blackwell Scientific Publications, 3rd edition 1995

Lecture Notes on Gynaecology
G Chamberlain and J Malvern, Blackwell Scientific Publications, 1996

Gynaecology Illustrated
A D T Govan, C Hodge and R Callander, Churchill Livingstone, 4th edition 1993 (also available as an International Student Edition)

Lecture Notes on Obstetrics
G Chamberlain, M Pearce and P Hamilton, Blackwell Scientific Publications, 1996

Obstetrics Illustrated
A W F Miller and R Callander, Churchill Livingstone, 1997 (also available as an International Student Edition)

EMQ PRACTICE EXAMINATION

200 questions: time allowed 3 hours

Theme: Colonic disorders

Options

A	Carcinoma of the caecum	E	Haemorrhoids
B	Carcinoma of the sigmoid colon	F	Irritable bowel syndrome
C	Colonic polyp	G	Sigmoid volvulus
D	Diverticulitis	H	Ulcerative colitis

For each patient listed below, choose the most appropriate diagnosis from the above list of options. Each option may be used once, more than once or not at all.

1. A 72-year-old man presents with increasing tiredness over a 2-year period. He has a microcytic anaemia and a mass in the right iliac fossa.

2. A 33-year-old woman consults you regarding symptoms of alternating diarrhoea and constipation associated with cramp-like abdominal pain.

3. A 76-year-old man presents with weight loss, pain on eating and abdominal distension. Plain abdominal X-ray films show the so called 'coffee bean' sign.

4. An 82-year-old woman presents to A & E with a distended abdomen. A plain abdominal x-ray film shows gross faecal loading in the colon and gas in the small bowel. The rectum is empty.

5. A 39-year-old woman presents with passage of bloodstained motions and mucus 5 times a day. Symptoms have persisted for over 1 month and are associated with weight loss. Barium enema shows no evidence of a colonic neoplasm, but a granular mucosa.

Theme: Causes of a sore mouth

Options

A	Antibiotic associated candidosis	G	Oral hairy leukoplakia
B	Burning mouth syndrome	H	Squamous cell carcinoma
C	Coated tongue	I	Systemic lupus erythematosus
D	Geographic tongue	J	Thrush
E	Iron deficiency	K	Trauma
F	Lichen planus	L	Vitamin B_{12} deficiency

For each of the following scenarios, choose the most likely diagnosis from the above list of options. Each option may be used once, more than once or not at all.

6. A 20-year-old woman who has become concerned about recurrent episodes of tongue soreness exacerbated by spicy foods and on looking at her tongue sees areas of erythematous depapillation which appear to move over the weeks.

7. A 65-year-old heavy smoker has had a long-standing increasingly painful ulcer on the lateral border of his tongue. He first noticed the ulcer 3 months ago and he is now having difficulty speaking.

8. A 55-year-old woman with a pruritic skin rash affecting her wrists and shins has also noticed oral soreness. On examination of her mouth she is found to have areas of white striae and ulceration affecting her tongue and buccal mucosa.

9. A 70-year-old woman is found to have a smooth, sore, red tongue with soreness and cracking at the corners of her mouth. She is undergoing investigation for a mass in her right iliac fossa.

10. A 23-year-old man with asthma complains of a sore mouth. On examination he is found to have an inflamed palate with white specks on it and a smooth red tongue.

Theme: Female urinary incontinence

Options

A	Anticholinergics	F	Midstream urinary sample
B	Clam cystoplasty	G	Pad test
C	Colposuspension operation	H	Pelvic floor exercise
D	Cystoscopy	I	Ultrasound scan of the bladder
E	Frequency/volume chart		

For each patient with urinary incontinence listed below, choose the next appropriate step of management from the above list of options. Each option may be used once, more than once or not at all.

11. A 23-year-old woman presents with a 3-day history of frequency, urgency and dysuria.

12. A 45-year-old woman had a vaginal bladder repair operation 2 weeks ago. Since then she frequently voids small volumes of clear urine and has developed increasing lower abdominal discomfort.

13. The diagnostic work-up of a 40-year-old woman has shown a mild degree of genuine stress incontinence.

Theme: Petechial rash in a child

Options

A   Acute lymphoblastic leukaemia
B   Henoch Schönlein purpura
C   Idiopathic thrombocytopaenic purpura
D   Meningococcaemia
E   Traumatic petechiae or ecchymoses

For each patient described below, choose the SINGLE most likely diagnosis from the above list of options. Each option may be used once, more than once or not at all.

14.   A 6-month-old baby presents with a history of paroxysmal cough of 4 days duration. The GP is concerned when examination reveals fine purpuric eruptions around her eyes and the neck. The baby has missed the DPT vaccination due to 'recurrent colds'.

15.   A 5-year-old girl develops colicky abdominal pain that is intermittent. The next day she has painful swelling of both her ankles and feet. Examination also reveals a palpable purpuric rash on the legs and larger confluent ecchymoses on the back of the thighs and the buttocks.

16.   A 12-year-old boy presents with fever of 12 hours duration when he develops headache and vomiting. The parents are concerned when he becomes rather lethargic and develops some spots on his limbs and chest. On examination he looks ill and is febrile, BP 90/45 mmHg, and a tachycardia at 140/min. He has poor capillary refill and sparse petechiae on upper and lower limbs.

17.   A 3-year-old girl has been 'unwell' for the past 10–14 days, being off colour, lethargic and with a poor appetite. Over the previous 48 hours she has developed bruises over her trunk and limbs. She is rather pale and has generalised enlargement of lymph nodes.

18.   A healthy 4-year-old boy develops bruises on his body over a period of 24 hours. This was also accompanied by a nose bleed for the first time. He has an upper respiratory infection with a low grade fever 2 weeks previously.

Theme: Acute abdomen

Options

A   Acute salpingitis
B   Adhesive small bowel obstruction
C   Appendicitis
D   Leaking aortic aneurysm
E   Mesenteric ischaemia
F   Pancreatitis
G   Perforated peptic ulcer
H   Ureteric colic

For each patient described below, choose the SINGLE most likely diagnosis from the above list of options. Each option may be used once, more than once or not at all.

19. A 60-year-old man with epigastric pain and brief collapse at home is now alert with some mild back pain and tachycardia.

20. A 45-year-old man has been taking ibuprofen for persistent abdominal pain. He has been brought to A & E after a sudden collapse, and an erect chest film shows gas under the diaphragm.

21. A 36-year-old woman has been brought to A & E by her husband with very severe left-sided abdominal pain. Her husband states that she has been pacing around the bedroom all night, unable to find a comfortable position, and the patient describes the pain as being 'worse than a labour pain'.

22. An 87-year-old woman is admitted with a rigid abdomen. A careful history reveals she has been having pain after meals and has stopped eating very much. Her blood gas assay reveals a metabolic acidosis. Her amylase level is within normal limits.

23. A 23-year-old woman presents with right iliac fossa pain for 4 days, associated with nausea but no vomiting. A dipstick urine test is normal and a careful history reveals an offensive vaginal discharge.

Theme: Otalgia

Options

A	Acute otitic barotrauma	I	Ramsay Hunt syndrome
B	Acute otitis externa	J	Squamous cell carcinoma of
C	Acute otitis media		the ear canal
D	Bell's palsy	K	Squamous cell carcinoma oF
E	Cervical spondylosis		the tongue
F	Furunculosis	L	Temporomandibular Joint
G	Malignant otitis externa		dysfunction
H	Myringitis bullosa		

For each of the following presentations, choose the most likely diagnosis from the above list of options. Each option may be used once, more than once or not at all.

24. A 70-year-old man presents with hearing loss, bloodstained discharge from the ear and facial paralysis.

25. A 6-year-old child complains of severe earache following an upper respiratory tract infection. She is unwell with fever and tachycardia. Examination shows a congested and bulging eardrum.

26. A 60-year-old man complains of sudden onset of right-sided earache with associated right-sided facial weakness. Examination reveals vesicles in the ipsilateral external auditory meatus and pharynx.

27. A 58-year-old woman has generalised discomfort and tenderness around and behind the ear. Movement of her neck is restricted and causes her to experience a similar pain.

28. A 68-year-old male lifelong cigarette smoker complains of worsening right sided earache, a sore tongue and difficulty talking.

Theme: Bleeding in pregnancy

Options

A	Abembryonic pregnancy	E	Ectopic pregnancy
B	Abruptio placenta	F	Insertio velamentosa
C	Cancer of the cervix	G	Molar pregnancy
D	Cervical erosion	H	Placenta praevia

For each of the following presentations, choose the most likely diagnosis from the above list of options. Each option may be used once, more than once or not at all.

29. A 20-year-old woman with a 7 weeks history of amenorrhoea with lower abdominal pain who fainted twice.

30. A 35-year-old para 5+1 with a painless bleeding of 200 ml at 35 weeks of pregnancy.

31. A women in advanced labour and normal vital signs with the fetal heart rate dropping steadily.

32. A woman presents at 16 weeks with the symphysial-fundal height measuring 20 cm and severe nausea, vomiting and heavy vaginal bleeding.

33. A 29-year-old para 3+2 with a history of intercourse the day before and painless dark brown bleeding of a teaspoonful of blood.

Theme: Small stature

Options

A   Congenital adrenal hyperplasia
B   Constitutional delay in puberty
C   Early onset puberty (idiopathic/ constitutional precocious puberty)
D   Familial (genetic) short stature
E   Growth hormone deficiency
F   Small-for-dates child (at birth)

For each patient described below, choose the SINGLE most likely diagnosis from the above options. Each option may be used once, more than once or not at all.

34.   A 12-year-old boy is referred because of not growing for the past 2 years. His classmates have overtaken him in stature though in the early years he was the tallest in the class and he needed changes of shoes and clothing very frequently at the time. History reveals that he developed pubic hair at 7–8 years of age and his voice 'changed' around the same time.

35.   A healthy 6-year-old has 'not grown' for the past 2–3 years. Born at term following a normal delivery he weighed 3.2 kg at birth. His initial growth has been satisfactory and developmental progress normal. The child's height is on 0.4th centile and the mid-parental centile for height lay between 50th and 75th centiles. Over the past year he has grown 2.3 cm.

36.   Parents are concerned about their 14-year-old son who has 'stopped growing' over the past 2–3 years and has been overtaken by the rest of his classmates. He is getting bullied and has dropped out of the school football team. Clinical examination was normal, the height lying on the 5th centile. No axillary or pubic hair is noted and the testicular volume is 2 ml. The bone age is reported as 11.4 years. Mid-parental centile for height is between the 25th and 50th centiles.

37. A 13-year-old white boy is referred by his GP because of short stature. He has always been the smallest in the class, but is an active child with no previous history of illness. Birth history was normal with weight of 3.7 kg at birth. His present height is 144 cm (4' 9") on the 9th centile and he has proceeded on this line for the last 5 years. The father is 5' 6" and mother 5' 1" tall. The bone age is 12.5 years.

38. A 13.5-year-old Asian girl is brought by her adoptive English parents because of their concern regarding her growth. She was adopted and brought to the U.K. at the age of 3 years. Her initial growth was normal, proceeding on the 25th to 50th centile until 11 years, and then slowed and has crossed to the 3rd centile. She had her menarche at 9.2 years.

Theme: Low urine output after surgery

Options

A   Acute tubular necrosis
B   Acute urinary retention
C   Blocked catheter
D   Chronic renal impairment
E   Intravascular depletion

For each of the following presentations, choose the most likely cause from the above list of options. Each option may be used once, more than once or not at all.

39.   An 80-year-old man who is normally hypertensive; postoperative day 1 following a right hemicolectomy. He has epidural analgesia and his blood pressure is 125/70 mmHg.

40.   A 65-year-old man has undergone a hernia repair as a day-case. He has not passed urine since the procedure and on examination a suprapubic mass is palpable.

41.   A 76-year-old man has undergone a TURP (transurethral resection of the prostate gland). In spite of irrigation his urine is heavily blood-stained and he is passing <20 ml/hour.

42.   A 35-year-old man has had a subtotal colectomy for ulcerative colitis. He has been given gentamicin antibiotic prophylaxis and diclofenac sodium for analgesia. It is the first postoperative day and his urine output has tailed off to <10 ml/hour.

Theme: Haematological conditions

Options

A   Acute lymphoblastic leukaemia
B   Acute myeloid leukaemia
C   Acute promyelocytic leukaemia
D   Chronic lymphocytic leukaemia
E   Chronic myeloid leukaemia
F   Hodgkin's lymphoma
G   Monoclonal gammopathy of undetermined significance
H   Multiple myeloma
I   Non-Hodgkin's lymphoma
J   Waldenström's macroglobulinaemia

For each of the following scenarios, choose the most likely diagnosis from the above list of options. Each option may be used once, more than once or not at all.

43. A 70-year-old retired farmer is found to have a peripheral blood lymphocytosis when a full blood count is taken after he presents to his general practitioner with herpes zoster.

44. A 60-year-old Afro-Caribbean man presents to his general practitioner with persistent bony pains. Initial blood investigations reveal an anaemia, raised ESR, urea and creatinine, and hypercalcaemia.

45. A pale four-year-old girl with recurrent infections and an ophthalmoplegia undergoes a full blood count and subsequent bone marrow investigation shows primitive pre-B lymphoblast cells.

46. An HIV-positive man on effective antiretroviral therapy presents with painless lymphadenopathy and fevers, drenching night sweats and weight loss.

47. A 50-year-old bank manager presents with tiredness, weight loss and sweating. He has noticed some visual disturbances. Examination reveals him to be pale and thin with splenomegaly. Haematological investigation reveals a massive neutrophilia with left shift but low neutrophil alkaline phosphatase score and a high serum vitamin B_{12} level.

Theme: Drugs in gynaecology

Options

A	Gonadotrophin releasing hormone analogues
B	Hormone replacement therapy
C	Mefenamic acid
D	Oral contraceptive pill
E	Progestogens
F	Tranexamic acid

In the management of gynaecological conditions, match the patients listed below with the most appropriate drug from the above list. Each option may be used once, more than once or not at all.

48. A 32-year-old woman with menorrhagia, planning a pregnancy.

49. A 17-year-old girl with irregular menstrual periods.

50. A 37-year-old smoker with primary dysmenorrhoea.

Theme: Paroxysmal cough in childhood

Options

A	Allergic rhinitis	D	Foreign body inhalation
B	Asthma	E	Gastro-oesophageal reflux
C	Cystic fibrosis	F	Pertussis

For each patient described below, choose the SINGLE most likely diagnosis from the above list of options. Each option may be used once, more than once or not at all.

51. A 2-year-old boy is seen with a history of a paroxysmal cough of sudden onset 2 days previously. He had been well before the onset and has been playing with his 5-year-old brother in the house. He also has a mild intermittent wheeze since the onset of the cough. He is not in any respiratory distress. Examination revealed diminution of air entry to the right lower chest posteriorly and the chest X-ray shows emphysema of the right lower lobe.

52. A 3-year-old girl has had a paroxysmal nocturnal cough intermittently for the past 6–8 months. She is well during the day with only a tendency to cough on exertion. The mother complains that each time she gets a cold 'it goes to her chest' and she has had frequent antibiotic treatment. There is a history of mild eczema. Clinically, except for a dry skin no abnormalities were noted.

53. An 18-month-old has had a paroxysmal nocturnal cough associated with a 'persistent cold' that has not cleared for several weeks. She starts to cough as she goes to sleep and may retch and vomit on some occasions. The cough is not severe during the day but she sounds 'rattly'. There is a strong history of atopy in the family.

54. A 5-week-old baby was admitted with cough and vomiting of 1 week's duration. Cough was paroxysmal sometimes associated with choking and transient cyanosis. Clinical examination reveals tachypnoea of 45/minute with good bilateral air entry and conducted sounds. The older sibling also has a less severe cough for the past 6 weeks and has not completed her immunisations.

Theme: Postoperative fever

Options

A   Basal lung collapse
B   CVP line infection
C   Subphrenic abscess
D   Urinary tract infection
E   Wound infection

For each patient described below, choose the SINGLE most likely diagnosis from the above list of options. Each option may be used once, more than once or not at all.

55. A 75-year-old man is discharged from the ICU after major abdominal surgery. He has a prolonged ileus, so TPN is commenced. On the 7th postoperative day he develops a temperature of 38.5°C.

56. An obese 45-year-old woman undergoes an open cholecystectomy for gallstones. She is slow to mobilise and on the second postoperative day develops a temperature of 37.9°C.

57. A 76-year-old man undergoes Hartmann's procedure for stercoral perforation. On the 8th postoperative day he develops a high spiking fever.

58. A 15-year-old boy undergoes an emergency appendicectomy for a perforated gangrenous appendix. On the 5th postoperative day he develops a temperature of 37.8°C and a thin serosanguineous discharge is noted on the wound dressing

Theme: Causes of oral ulceration

Options

A	Behçet's disease	G	Reiter's syndrome
B	Crohn's disease	H	Shingles
C	Erythema multiforme	I	Squamous cell carcinoma
D	Lichen planus	J	Syphilis
E	Oral mucositis	K	Systemic lupus erythematosus
F	Recurrent oral ulceration	L	Ulcerative colitis

For each of the following scenarios, choose the most likely diagnosis from the above list of options. Each option may be used once, more than once or not at all.

59. A 40-year-old HIV-positive patient presents with a 2-day history of pain affecting the right side of his face, followed by a vesicular rash affecting both his midface and the right side of his palate.

60. A 15-year-old schoolgirl presents with a 2-year history of up to five painful oral ulcers occurring at intervals of 1–2 months. She is otherwise well.

61. A 25-year-old Turkish man has been suffering from recurrent orogenital ulceration. He is now complaining of floaters affecting his vision, increasing acne-like lesions and joint pains.

62. A 30-year-old woman given oral trimethoprim for a urinary tract infection develops discrete target-like lesions on her skin with severe oral ulceration and crusting of the lips.

63. A 35-year-old man returns from an extended period of overseas travel and develops a small papule on his upper lip which rapidly breaks down into a large painless indurated ulcer.

Theme: Investigations for suspected malignant disease in gynaecology

Options

A   CT abdomen and pelvis
B   Cytology
C   D&C alone
D   Diagnostic laparoscopy
E   Examination under anaesthesia and representative biopsies
F   Hysteroscopy alone
G   Hysteroscopy and D&C
H   Pelvic ultrasound scan

For each patient listed below, choose the investigation of FIRST choice from the above list of options. Each option may be used once, more than once or not at all.

64. A 65-year-old obese, diabetic and hypertensive woman presents with two recent episodes of postmenopausal bleeding.

65. A 59-year-old woman noticed loss of appetite, constipation and a swollen abdomen. She had a pelvic ultrasound scan which showed cystic ovaries.

66. A 38-year-old woman attends for a smear test 10 years after the previous one. On speculum examination the cervix looks irregular in shape and bleeds easily on touch.

Theme: Sepsis in childhood

Options

A	*Escherichia coli*	E	*Pseudomonas aeruginosa*
B	Group B streptococcus	F	*Salmonella typhimurium*
C	*Mycoplasma pneumoniae*	G	*Staphylococcus aureus*
D	*Pneumocystis carinii*	H	*Staphylococcus epidermidis*

For each patient described below, choose the single most likely causative organism from the above list of options. Each option may be used once, more than once or not at all.

67. An 8-year-old girl treated for acute lymphoblastic leukaemia who is in remission develops high fever 3 days after the last course of chemotherapy. Otherwise she was asymptomatic and clinically no focus of sepsis was found. The WBC was 1100/ml with a neutrophil count of 650. The blood culture taken via the portacath grew a pure growth of an organism.

68. A 9-year-old girl originally diagnosed at the age of 7 months with cystic fibrosis has had multiple admissions with recurrent chest infections over the past 2 years needing intravenous antibiotic therapy. There has been rapid deterioration of her lung function during this period with the persistence of an organism in the sputum that was difficult to eradicate.

69. A 14-year-old Nigerian boy presents with fever and painful swelling of his left knee joint soon after returning from a holiday in Nigeria. He has sickle cell disease and during the last week of his stay in Africa developed an acute gastro-enteritis which is now settling. Aspiration of the joint yielded a purulent fluid that grew an organism.

70. A 2-day-old baby is transferred from the maternity unit because of increasing respiratory distress, lethargy and poor feeding. The delivery was normal at 37 weeks with no immediate problems. Clinically the baby appears ill with peripheral circulatory failure and respiratory distress. The chest X-ray reveals bilateral inflammatory changes. The blood culture and the mother's high vaginal swab grew the same organism.

71. A 12-year-old develops fever with rigors and painful swelling of the right ankle and was seen in hospital 3 days later. There was a tender swelling of the lower leg and ankle with marked tenderness. Investigation revealed a leucocytosis with a high neutrophil count, and high ESR and CRP levels. X-rays of the ankle and lower tibia are normal. A blood culture grew an organism.

72. A 10-month-old baby develops high fever with rigors and vomiting and has stopped feeding. At presentation she is in shock with cold peripheries needing fluid resuscitation. She is commenced on antibiotics immediately as septic shock is suspected. Her blood and urine cultures both grew the same organism. Subsequent imaging revealed bilateral vesico-ureteric reflux.

Theme: Thyroid malignancies

Options

A	Anaplastic
B	Follicular
C	Lymphoma
D	Medullary
E	Papillary

For each description below, select the most appropriate type of thyroid malignancy from the above list of options. Each option may be used once, more than once or not at all.

73. Rare, and presents as an enlarging firm painless mass in elderly women.

74. Associated with the multiple endocrine neoplasias.

75. Affects middle-aged patients, has a good prognosis.

76. Associated with raised plasma calcitonin level.

Theme: Orofacial manifestations of systemic disease

Options

A	ACE inhibitor therapy	G	Dietary allergy
B	Beta blocker therapy	H	HIV disease
C	Bulimia nervosa	I	Mumps
D	C1 esterase deficiency	J	Nifedipine therapy
E	Chronic alcohol use	K	Sarcoidosis
F	Crohn's disease	L	Sjögren's syndrome

For each of the following scenarios, choose the most likely diagnosis from the above list of options. Each option may be used once, more than once or not at all.

77. A 65-year-old man with hypertension develops gingival hyperplasia.

78. An otherwise healthy 13-year-old boy presents with recurrent episodes of facial and tongue swelling and abdominal pain. His father has had similar episodes.

79. A 70-year-old woman presents with recurrent episodes of parotid swelling. She complains of difficulty talking and speaking and her eyes feel gritty on waking in the morning.

80. A thin 18-year-old girl has bilateral parotid swelling with thickened calluses on the dorsum of her hand.

81. A 40-year-old man with marked weight loss over the preceding 6 months has bilateral white, vertically corrugated lesions on the lateral surfaces of the tongue.

Theme: Management of labour

Options

A	CTG monitoring
B	Emergency caesarean section
C	Fetal blood sampling
D	Hydration
E	Instrumental vaginal delivery
F	Oxygen supply
G	Ultrasound scan

For each patient listed below, choose the most appropriate step of management from the options above. Each option may be used once, more than once or not at all.

82. A 31-year-old obese woman presents in early labour. On vaginal examination the midwife found an 'empty' pelvis.

83. A primiparous woman is admitted at 38 weeks gestation in early labour. At vaginal examination the cervix is found to be 2 cm dilated and thick meconium seen. The CTG is abnormal.

84. A primiparous woman is fully dilated for 3 hours and actively pushing for 1 hour. The fetal head is in occipito-posterior position 4 cm below the ischial spine.

85. A multiparous woman is in advanced labour and the CTG is showing variable decelerations.

86. A primiparous women presents in early labour. The fetus is known to be small for gestational age.

Theme: Chronic diarrhoea in infancy and childhood

Options

A	Cystic fibrosis
B	Giardiasis
C	Gluten enteropathy
D	Hirschsprung disease
E	Milk protein intolerance.
F	Toddler diarrhoea
G	Ulcerative colitis or chronic inflammatory bowel disease

For each patient described below, choose the SINGLE most likely diagnosis from the above options. Each option may be used once, more than once or not at all.

87. A 15-year-old boy has had abdominal pain and diarrhoea intermittently for the past 2 years. Recently the frequency of his complaints has increased with passage of blood and mucus in the stools and loss of weight. He also suffers from intermittent fever and joint pains and on examination is noted to have erythema nodosum lesions on his shins.

88. An 18-month-old boy has had frequent loose motions for the past 6–8 months. Frequency varied from 4 to 8 stools per day, loose to watery. No blood or mucus but has undigested vegetable matter in the stool. He feeds well and is gaining weight satisfactorily. Repeatedly, stool examinations and investigations are normal.

89. A 7-month-old girl has been passing large offensive stools since 3 months of age. She feeds well but her weight has gradually fallen across the centiles from the 75th to the 9th. She has had persistent 'chestiness' needing frequent antibiotics.

90. A 1-year-old girl presents because of 'failure to thrive' and diarrhoea. Having initially grown well the child has gradually dropped below the 2nd centile in weight over the last 6 months. Clinically she is wasted, anaemic and has abdominal distension. Stools are described as 'large, loose, offensive and difficult to flush'. An IgA anti-endomysial antibody in serum was positive.

91. A 3-month-old male infant presents with abdominal distension and alternating diarrhoea and constipation since 4 weeks of age. The stools vary between hard small pellets and loose motions with mucus. There is a history of delay in passage of meconium after birth of 3 days.

Theme: Biliary tract

Options

A   An acutely raised amylase
B   Left-sided pleural effusion
C   ERCP – endoscopic retrograde cholangio-pancreatography
D   Persistently elevated amylase
E   Raised alkaline phosphatase and bilirubin
F   None of the above

From the list above, choose the most appropriate option to match the statements below. Each option may be used once, more than once or not at all.

92.   Can remove a stone from the common bile duct.

93.   Associated with pseudocyst formation.

94.   Commonly caused by stone in the common bile duct.

95.   A prognostic indicator in acute pancreatitis.

96.   May cause pancreatitis.

Theme: Facial appearance

Options

A	Acne rosacea	G	Mitral stenosis
B	Addison's disease	H	Peutz-Jeghers syndrome
C	Chloasma	I	Rhinophyma
D	Discoid lupus erythematosus	J	Sarcoidosis
E	Lupus pernio	K	Seborrhoeic dermatitis
F	Lupus vulgaris	L	Systemic lupus erythematosus

For each of the following scenarios, choose the most likely cause for the facial rash described from the above list of options. Each option may be used once, more than once or not at all.

97. A 25-year-old man with excessive dandruff and a pruritic erythematous rash affecting his eyebrows, ears, scalp and lateral margins of the nose.

98. A 35-year-old woman with a malar butterfly rash complains of a dry mouth and joint pains.

99. A 40-year-old woman with a diffuse, purple-red infiltration of the nose and cheeks. She has had a persistent dry cough, mild dyspnoea, weight loss and malaise for over a year. Chest examination appears normal.

100. A patient presents to the A & E department with recurrent colicky abdominal pain. There are a number of small brownish-black macules affecting the perioral skin and oral mucosa.

101. A 45-year-old man presents with a persistent reddish papulopustular rash affecting the cheeks, nose, forehead and chin. The nose appears bulbous and craggy.

Theme: Causes for amenorrhoea

Options

A	Absent uterus
B	Constitutional
C	Imperforate hymen
D	Prolactinoma
E	Sheehan's syndrome
F	XO-karyotype

For each of the scenarios listed below, choose the most likely cause from the above options. Each option may be used once, more than once or not at all.

102. A 16-year-old girl with normal secondary characteristics gives a history of cyclical abdominal pain.

103. An asymptomatic 17-year-old girl with normal secondary characteristics and normal endocrine results has a negative progesterone challenge test.

104. A 35-year-old woman had a normal vaginal delivery followed by a massive postpartum haemorrhage.

105. An 18-year-old woman has a short stature and absent secondary sexual characteristics.

Theme: Fits and faints in children

Options

A   Benign paroxysmal vertigo
B   Breath-holding attacks (cyanotic spells)
C   Complex partial seizure
D   Congenital heart block
E   Reflex anoxic seizure (pallid spells)
F   Supraventricular tachycardia
G   Syncope

For each patient described below, choose the SINGLE most likely diagnosis from the above list of options. Each option may be used once, more than once or not at all.

106. A 10-year-old had three episodes of loss of consciousness, the first two at school and the last on a shopping outing at a crowded summer sale. She was well prior to the attacks (all having occurred when she had been standing among a crowd). She had felt dizzy, nauseated and become pale and sweaty before losing consciousness for about 2 minutes. There was no incontinence but twitching of the fingers was noted. On recovery she felt tired.

107. A 2.5-year-old had three episodes of vomiting and sudden onset of ataxia over the past 6 months. The attacks were rather short (5–10 minutes) but during which he appeared frightened and pale and had to lie down. After the attack he was back to normal. It was mentioned that he keeps his eyes down or closed when travelling by car or lift.

108. A 15-month-old girl has had recurrent episodes of loss of consciousness precipitated by temper tantrums. She is developmentally within normal limits. When upset she starts with a shrill cry, goes blue and floppy, losing consciousness for about 1 minute during which a few jerky movement of limbs may occur.

109. A 7-year-old boy has had four episodes of loss of consciousness over the past 6 months. Two occurred in the morning soon after he woke up when he was noticed to be in a 'dreamlike state' with his head turned to the right and doing 'pill rolling' movements with his hand. This was followed by loss of posture and a generalised seizure lasting 3–4 minutes.

110. A 3-year-old with history of five attacks of loss of consciousness associated with minor trauma such as knocking of his head or injury to his finger. He becomes pale, loses consciousness and goes floppy, sometimes twitching slightly. During one attack he had a heart rate of 30 beats per minute which rapidly recovered. He regained consciousness rapidly each time.

Theme: Hair loss

Options

A	Alopecia areata	G	Lupus erythematosus
B	Androgenetic alopecia	H	Malnutrition
C	Colchicine	I	Scalp ringworm
D	Hypothyroidism	J	Secondary syphilis
E	Iron deficiency	K	Telogen effluvium
F	Lichen planus	L	Traumatic

For each of the following scenarios, choose the most likely diagnosis from the above list of options. Each option may be used once, more than once or not at all.

111. A 55-year-old woman is complaining about patchy hair loss with localised areas of erythema, scaling and scarring affecting the scalp. She has a sore mouth and a skin rash affecting the flexor surfaces of her wrists and shins.

112. A 20-year-old man presents with sharply defined non-erythematous patches of baldness on his scalp. His eyebrows and beard are also affected and examination of the individual hairs show that they taper towards the scalp.

113. Three months after experiencing a severe illness with high fevers an 18-year-old man notices excessive numbers of hairs in his hairbrush and on his pillow.

114. A 50-year-old woman notices some diffuse thinning of her hair with bitemporal recession.

115. A 65-year-old woman presents with thinning hair, loss of the outer third of her eyebrows and lethargy.

Theme: Investigations in pregnancy

Options

A	24 hour urine protein excretion
B	Amniocentesis
C	Bile acids
D	Doppler ultrasound of the umbilical artery
E	Glucose tolerance test
F	Kleihauer test

For each patient listed below, choose the investigation of FIRST choice from the above list of options. Each option may be used once, more than once or not at all.

116. A rhesus-negative woman has a significant antepartum haemorrhage at 29 weeks gestation.

117. A 29-year-old primiparous woman presents at 35 weeks with itching.

118. A 35-year-old multiparous woman is admitted with a blood pressure of 160/95 mmHg and 1+ protein excretion in the urine dipstick test.

119. A 27-year-old woman has a reduced symphysial-fundal height at clinical examination. A subsequently arranged ultrasound scan reveals intrauterine growth restriction.

120. The triple test of a 25-year-old woman has shown that her baby is at increased risk of having Down's syndrome.

Theme: Investigation of neuromuscular disease

Options:

A	Blood glucose	E	ECG
B	Chromosomal analysis	F	EEG
C	Creatine phosphokinase	G	MRI of brain
D	CT scan	H	Muscle biopsy

For each patient below, choose the MOST appropriate investigation from the above list of options. Each option may be used once, more than once or not at all.

121. A 12-hour-old baby stops sucking and starts to have generalised seizures. The delivery had been normal at 41 weeks with good Apgar scores and the baby weighed 2.3 kg. No other physical or clinical abnormality is noted.

122. A 3-year-old boy presented because of delayed walking. He took his first steps alone at just over 2 years, but his progress is not satisfactory as he still finds it difficult to climb stairs or to get up from the floor when he 'climbs on his legs'. Manipulation and hand-eye co-ordination is normal.

123. A 4-year-old boy has over the past 3 months become increasingly 'clingy' and miserable with intermittent episodes of vomiting. His mother notices that he loses his balance and has started bumping into things. There is no history of fits. Clinically he is ataxic with exaggeration of deep reflexes and ?early papilloedema.

124. A 5-month-old girl has over the past 4–6 weeks started having episodes of staring and head nodding sometimes with jerking of all four limbs. The frequency of these attacks has increased to 10–20 times a day. Parents feel that the baby has stopped smiling and attempting to turn over.

125. The newborn baby of a 32-year-old primiparous mother is noted to be markedly hypotonic at the initial examination at 24 hours. The baby fed poorly and examination also indicated presence of single palmar creases. The mother's antenatal ultrasound examination has not picked up any abnormality and the 'dual test' for Down's syndrome gives the probability as 1 in 1024.

126. An 11-year-old girl presents after sudden loss of consciousness that lasted about 3 minutes. Clinical examination soon afterwards reveals a pulse rate of 30 beats per minute with an apical short systolic murmur. There was no previous history. Chest X-ray reveals an enlarged heart shadow.

Theme: Causes of dysphagia

Options

A	Achalasia	F	Myasthenia gravis
B	Bronchial carcinoma	G	Oesophageal candidosis
C	Carcinoma of the oesophagus	H	Pharyngeal pouch
D	Chronic benign stricture	I	Plummer-Vinson syndrome
E	Left atrial hypertrophy	J	Reflux oesophagitis

For each patient below, choose the most likely diagnosis from the above list of options. Each option may be used once, more than once or not at all.

127. A 50-year-old obese woman complains of a burning retrosternal discomfort after eating and on lying down. She has also noticed excessive salivation and wheezing when she lies down to sleep.

128. A 35-year-old housewife has noticed progressively worsening difficulty swallowing over several years. She has been troubled by regurgitation of undigested food and halitosis, and suffers fits of coughing on lying flat.

129. A 45-year-old pale woman complains that food is sticking in the back of her throat. On examination she is found to have spoon-shaped nails, a smooth tongue and angular cheilitis.

130. A 65-year-old man complains of difficulty in swallowing. He finds that the first mouthful of food is easy to swallow but thereafter he has increasing difficulty in swallowing until he regurgitates undigested food. He also notices a neck swelling.

131. A 60-year-old woman complains of difficulty swallowing. On examination she is found to have a prominent malar flush, an irregularly irregular pulse, an elevated jugular venous pressure and on auscultation has a rumbling, long, low-pitched, mid-diastolic murmur best heard in the left lateral position in expiration.

Theme: Health benefits from contraceptives

Options

A	Barrier methods
B	Combined oral contraceptive pill
C	Copper intrauterine device
D	Depo-Provera injections
E	Mirena coil
F	Natural methods
G	Progesterone only pill
H	Sterilisation

Match each of the following with the most appropriate contraceptive from the above list of options.

132. Reduction of the risks of endometrial and ovarian cancer.

133. Reduction of sexually transmitted diseases.

134. Improvement of the quality of breast milk postpartum.

135. Improvement of primary dysmenorrhoea.

136. Recognized treatment of menorrhagia in smokers over the age of 35 years.

Theme: Investigation of neonatal jaundice

Options

A   ABO haemolytic disease of new-born
B   Biliary atresia
C   G6PD deficiency
D   Galactosaemia
E   Hypothyroidism
F   Neonatal hepatitis
G   Neonatal sepsis

From the above list of options, choose the MOST likely diagnosis for each of the following clinical presentations. Each option may be used once, more than once or not at all.

137. A 5-day-old baby born at 36 weeks weighing 3 kg becomes lethargic and has gone off feeds. The mild icterus noted on the 3rd day has deepened and clinically the baby looks ill. Investigations were as follows: WBC 18000, neutrophils 13500. Na 131 mmol, Urea 9.8 mmol, CRP 80, S Bilirubin 220 micromol. Art pH 7.26, base deficit −14.2 mmol.

138. A 4-day-old baby is noted to have mild icterus when seen by the midwife in the morning. Birth was at 40 weeks by normal delivery, weight being 3.850 kg. She was breast fed and had been feeding well. The baby was brought to hospital 8 hours later as her jaundice had rapidly worsened. Investigations were: serum bilirubin 380 micromol (95% unconjugated), Hb 7.2 g/l, both mother and baby are Group A Rh +ve. The parents are of Mediterranean origin.

139. A 6-day-old infant develops vomiting, followed by a prolonged convulsion. She had been irritable and lethargic. Examination revealed an ill infant with moderate jaundice and significant liver enlargement. Investigations were: serum bilirubin 180 micromol, blood glucose 1.0 mmol, Hb 14 gm%, WBC 13000, normal differential count, CRP 15, ALT 80 units, GGT 120 units, urine reducing substances positive (Clinitest).

140. A 6-week-old baby presents with persistent jaundice since birth. The mother delivered the baby as an emergency, having recently arrived in the UK from an Asian country. The birth weight was 3.4 kg, with normal Apgar scores. The baby is snuffly and develops a cough. Examination: respiratory rate 50/min, liver 3 cm below costal margin. Investigations: total bilirubin 120 mmol, conjugated bilirubin 65 mmol, free thyroxine 14.2 pmol, TSH 6.2 uIU, ALT 70 units, GGT 110 units, alk phosphatase 800 units. The chest X-ray was clear but the right humerus showed a periostial reaction.

Theme: Pruritus

Options

A	Chronic renal failure	G	Lymphoma
B	Dermatitis herpetiformis	H	Old age
C	Eczema	I	Polycythaemia
D	Iron deficiency	J	Pregnancy
E	Lichen planus	K	Scabies
F	Liver disease	L	Thyroid disease

For each of the patients below, choose the most likely cause for their pruritus. Each option may be used once, more that once or not at all.

141. A 55-year-old woman presents complaining of oral soreness exacerbated by spicy foods and a pruritic, cutaneous rash principally affecting her shins and the flexor surfaces of her wrists.

142. A 30-year-old man presents with groups of small intensely itchy vesicles affecting the skin on his knees, elbows, buttocks and scalp.

143. A 55-year-an old woman presents with recurrent headaches, intermittent visual disturbances, angina and Raynaud's phenomenon. She has been troubled by a generalized itch that is worse after a hot bath. Examination reveals splenomegaly and bruises.

144. A 19-year-old man is seen in clinic with painless cervical lymphadenopathy initially noticed by his girlfriend. He has been feeling lethargic for some time with night sweats and itchy skin.

145. A 70-year-old woman complains of generalized itch, tiredness and shortness of breath on exercise. On examination she appears pale, and thin with brittle, spoon-shaped nails.

Theme: Convulsion in pregnancy

Options:

A	Cerebral infarction	G	Hypoglycaemia
B	Cerebral vein thrombosis	H	Hyponatraemia
C	Drug and alcohol withdrawal	I	Pseudoepilepsy
D	Eclampsia	J	Thrombotic thrombocytopenic
E	Epilepsy		purpura
F	Gestational epilepsy		

For each patient listed below, choose the most likely cause of convulsion from the above list of options. Each option may be used once, more than once or not at all.

146. A 39-year-old hypertensive multiparous woman who smokes 25 cigarettes per day.

147. An 18-year-old primiparous women in early labour who was induced for a sudden rise of blood pressure.

148. A 25-year-old woman who has been on methadone for the past 3 weeks.

149. A 27-year-old woman who has had two second-trimester pregnancy losses in the past and a deep vein thrombosis outside pregnancy.

Theme: Heart disease in childhood

Options

A   Aortic stenosis
B   AV septal defect
C   Dilated cardiomyopathy
D   Innocent murmur
E   Patent ductus arteriosis
Γ   Tetralogy of Fallot

For each group of clinical features described below, choose the SINGLE most likely diagnosis from the above list of options. Each option may be used once, more than once or not at all.

150. A 4-week-old baby needed ventilatory support for 4 days and is weaned off to air. Two days later he becomes tachypnoeic with poor feeding and has three episodes of apnoea. There is an increase in weight. Clinically peripheral perfusion is poor and in the CVS, the precordium is active and the peripheral pulses are bounding. A loud systolic murmur is heard in the pulmonary area. Chest X-ray shows pulmonary oedema.

151. A 9-month-old recovers from a respiratory infection but increasingly gets breathless first on exertion and subsequently at rest. He is tachycardic. The apex beat was on the left anterior axillary line in the 6th intercostal space. Liver is 3 cm below costal margin. A gallop rhythm was present with a pansystolic murmur at the apex. ECG shows widened QRS complexes and LV preponderance. Chest X-ray shows gross cardiomegaly.

152. A 16-week-old baby is noted to get 'blue discoloration' of the arms and legs intermittently with no associated dyspnoea. The baby was pink at birth and subsequent clinical examinations were normal. On examination the baby's growth was found to be within normal limits. No cyanosis is noted. Peripheral pulses are normal. No cardiac enlargement. A thrill is felt in the pulmonary area with a rough ejection systolic murmur best heard in the same area. P2 was single and quiet. ECG shows RV hypertrophy with a right QRS axis. CXR shows oligaemic lungs. O_2 saturation is 89–92% in air.

153. An 8-year-old boy develops faintness associated with central chest pain while playing football. This has recently been restricting him due to discomfort but he has not been breathless. On examination peripheral pulses felt well. BP 126/78 mmHg. Hyperactive apex. Systolic thrill felt suprasternally. Harsh systolic murmur at apex and aortic area. ECG: left ventricular hypertrophy.

154. A 4-month-old baby with breathlessness and failure to thrive. A cardiac murmur was first noted around 6 weeks of age. Not cyanosed but tachypnoeic and tachycardic. Hyperdynamic apex beat. Loud P2. Loud pansystolic murmur at left sternal edge. ECG: RA enlargement, QRS +230, RV hypertrophy. CXR : Enlarged heart, prominent pulmonary artery and pulmonary plethora.

Theme: Findings on physical examination

Options

A	Argyll Robertson pupil	G	Lambert-Eaton myasthenic
B	Bronchial carcinoma		syndrome
C	Cirrhosis	H	Multiple sclerosis
D	Cystic fibrosis	I	Myasthenia gravis
E	Holmes-Adie syndrome	J	Pericardial effusion
F	Horner's syndrome		

For each patient's clinical presentation below, choose the single most likely diagnosis from the above list. Each option may be used once, more than once or not at all.

155. A young woman has noticed increasing muscle weakness, double vision and difficulty swallowing. Ptosis, ophthalmoplegia, dysarthria and distal muscle weakness with normal reflexes are found on clinical examination.

156. A 35-year-old male intravenous drug user with finger clubbing, leukonychia, palmar erythema and gynaecomastia.

157. A woman is found to have a moderately dilated left pupil which is poorly reactive to light. She has absent knee and ankle reflexes.

158. A patient in the immediate postoperative recovery period from a coronary artery bypass graft complains of increasing chest discomfort, dysphagia, hoarseness, dyspnoea with muffled heart sounds and an absent apical impulse on examination.

159. Haemoptysis in a 55-year-old cigarette smoker in whom the finger nails show an exaggerated longitudinal curve with loss of the angle between the nail and the nail bed.

Theme: Diagnosis in gynaecology

Options

A	Cancer of the endometrium	E	Pelvic inflammatory disease
B	Irritable bowel syndrome	F	Ruptured ovarian cyst
C	Ovarian cancer	G	Torsion of an ovarian cyst
D	Pelvic endometriosis		

Which would be the most likely diagnosis from the above list of options in the patients listed below? Each option may be used once, more than once or not at all.

160. An 18-year-old woman who is not sexually active presents at mid-cycle with acute onset of lower abdominal pain, which resolves 6 hours after admission.

161. A 24-year-old woman in a stable relationship presents in the clinic with a 1-year history of lower abdominal pain, deep dyspareunia and an inability to conceive.

162. A 49-year-old woman noticed an increase in abdominal girth alongside with constipation and weight loss.

163. A 23-year-old woman had a diagnostic laparoscopy for recurrent lower abdominal pain, which showed normal pelvic organs. High vaginal swab and endocervical swabs were negative.

Theme: Drug treatment in childhood

Options

A	Co-trimoxazole	F	Prostaglandin E
B	Dexamethasone	G	Rifampicin
C	Digoxin	H	Sodium valproate
D	Enalapril	I	Vancomycin
E	Indomethacin	J	Vigabatrin

For each patient below choose the SINGLE most appropriate medication from the above list. Each option may be used once, more than once or not at all.

164. An 18-month-old child known to be HIV positive has had a chronic cough of over 3 months duration. Chest X-ray showed bilateral infiltrates and a granular pattern and tracheal aspirates are positive for *Pneumocystis carinii*.

165. An 11-month-old presents with multiple fits, mostly absences, and a few major tonic /clonic fits within a period of 2 months. Clinically there is an ash leaf skin lesion but no neurological deficit. The CT scan shows three small subependymal tubers.

166. A 2-month-old baby develops increasing breathlessness, cough and poor feeding. Examination reveals a baby failing to thrive and tachypnoeic. There is no cyanosis. The apex is hyperdynamic. A loud pansystolic murmur and a short mid-diastolic rumble are heard over the precordium. P2 is loud and split. Liver is 4 cm below the costal margin. Has been on frusemide and spironolactone with no improvement.

167. Two siblings aged 5 and 9 years respectively of a child with a confirmed case of meningococcal disease present for prophylactic antibiotic therapy.

168. A 10-day-old baby born at 32 weeks needs IPPV for 6 days and is successfully weaned off when she redevelops respiratory distress. Clinically the pulses are bounding and there is a loud continuous murmur in the pulmonary area. Fluid restriction and diuretics are not helpful.

169. A 6-month-old baby presents with frequent attacks of head nodding with flexion of limbs over the past 6 weeks. The baby has become more lethargic and appears to have regressed in his activities and stopped smiling. An EEG shows a chaotic high-voltage non-synchronous pattern.

170. A 2-week-old neonate born at 28 weeks and having a central line becomes ill and 'septic'. Blood culture grows multi-resistant *Staphylococcus aureus* . The baby had been on penicillin and gentamicin for 5 days post-natally for prolonged rupture of membranes.

Theme: Autoantibodies

Options

A   Anti smooth muscle antibody
B   Anti-DS DNA
C   Anti-Jo 1
D   Anti-La
E   Anti-RNP
F   Anti-Ro
G   Anti-Scl 70
H   Centromere staining pattern of antinuclear antibodies
I   Homogeneous staining pattern of anti nuclear antibodies
J   Rheumatoid factor

For each patient's clinical presentation below, choose the single most significantly associated autoantibody from the list above. Each response may be used once, more than once or not at all.

171. A neonate born with congenital heart block.

172. A patient who has been receiving isoniazid for tuberculosis develops a photosensitive rash, oral ulcers and pleurisy.

173. A 50-year-old jaundiced woman with xanthelasma, hepatosplenomegaly and a raised alkaline phosphatase on liver function tests. Liver biopsy shows granulomas around the bile ducts.

174. A patient with dysphagia, thin tapering fingers with calcified subcutaneous nodules, and Raynaud's phenomenon.

175. An elderly woman with severe symmetrical metacarpophalangeal joint and wrist arthritis and subcutaneous nodules affecting the extensor surfaces of her elbows.

Theme: Adverse drug effects

Options

A	Amiodarone	F	Digoxin
B	Amphotericin	G	Methotrexate
C	Ampicillin	H	Nifedipine
D	Bleomycin	I	Phenytoin
E	Cyclosporin	J	Retinoids

For each medication above, choose the most likely associated drug adverse effect from the list below. Each option may be used once, more than once or not at all.

176. Gynaecomastia.

177. Severe mucositis.

178. Dry mucous membranes.

179. Blue-grey discoloration in sun-exposed areas of the skin.

180. Hirsuitism.

Theme: Arterial pulses

Options

A	Absent	E	Jerky
B	Alternans	F	Paradoxical
C	Bisferiens	G	Slow rising
D	Collapsing		

For the list below, choose the arterial pulse characteristic which is likely to be encountered on physical examination. Each option may be used once, more than once or not at all.

181. Aortic regurgitation.

182. Severe cardiac tamponade.

183. Severe left ventricular failure.

184. Aortic stenosis.

185. Takayasu's arteritis.

Theme: Psychiatric presentations

Options

A	Agitated depression	F	Hyperkinetic disorder
B	Bipolar affective disorder	G	Panic disorder
C	Cyclothymia	H	Schizophrenia
D	Dysthymia	I	Seasonal affective disorder
E	Generalised anxiety disorder	J	Somatization disorder

For each patient's clinical presentation below, choose the single most likely diagnosis from the list above. Each response may be used once, more than once or not at all.

186. A 25-year-old junior advertising executive who has previously suffered from depression is noticed by work colleagues to have become socially and sexually disinhibited and euphoric, and has started a number of unrealistic work projects that he has not concentrated on. He is overactive, has pressure of speech and is not sleeping.

187. A middle-aged housewife presents with depressed affect, loss of libido, amenorrhoea, reduced appetite and early morning wakening at the start of winter. Similar symptoms occurred at the same time last year and resolved in summer.

188. A 25-year-old woman repeatedly attends her local A & E department and general practitioner's surgery with frequently recurring different symptoms, demanding assessment and refusing to accept reassurance despite consistently negative results.

Theme: Red eyes

Options

A	Acute angle closure glaucoma	F	Scleritis
B	Allergic conjunctivitis	G	Subconjunctival haemorrhage
C	Anterior uveitis	H	Ulcerative keratitis
D	Bacterial conjunctivitis	I	Viral conjunctivitis
E	Chlamydial conjunctivitis		

For each patient's clinical presentation below, choose the single most likely diagnosis from the list above. Each option may be used once, more than once or not at all.

189. A young man with lower back pain complains of recurrent episodes of photophobia with painful, watering, red eyes and reduced visual acuity.

190. A patient complains of difficulty opening the eyes on waking with a purulent discharge and discomfort from both eyes. The conjunctivae are inflamed. There is no loss of visual acuity

191. A 55-year-old man describes sudden onset of severe pain in one eye associated with vomiting coming on in the evening. He has noticed impaired vision and haloes around lights. Examination reveals an inflamed and tender eye with a fixed and semi-dilated pupil.

192. A 35-year-old dentist complains of a painful, red eye and photophobia. There is a watery discharge. Fluorescein drops demonstrate dendritic corneal ulceration.

193. A 30-year-old woman with recovering from an upper respiratory tract infection presents with a dramatically red but painless eye.

Theme: Disorders of the knee joint

Options

A	Anterior cruciate ligament injury	F	Osteosarcoma of the proximal tibia
B	Gout	G	Patella bursitis
C	Meniscal injury	H	Patella fracture
D	Osgood Schlatter's disease	I	Rheumatoid arthritis
E	Osteoarthritis	J	Septic arthritis

For each patient below select the ONE most likely diagnosis. Each option may be used once, more than once or not at all.

194. A 33-year-old nurse was running for the bus when she tripped and fell over an uneven paving slab. She felt something crack and afterwards was unable to bear weight on the leg. In A & E considerable bruising around the knee is noted. She is unable to lift her leg off the couch.

195. A 13-year-old boy presents to his GP with a 6-month history of pain and swelling at the front of his knee. His symptoms are exacerbated by exercise and relieved by rest. There is now a prominent lump anteriorly over the proximal tibia. There is no specific history of trauma. His friend has recently been treated for leukaemia.

196. A 55-year-old ex-footballer presents to his GP with a long history of aches and pains in various joints. He has had previous meniscectomies of both knees and since he took part in a charity match last weekend he has been aware of considerable pain and swelling in his right knee. He can barely walk. Examination confirms a large tense effusion within the joint and significant restriction in joint movement. He is otherwise well.

197. A 55-year-old publican presents to his GP with a 24-hour history of acute pain and swelling in his left knee. He has been unable to sleep. Examination confirmed a large effusion in his knee and considerable tenderness. He is known to have a recent history of congestive cardiac failure but no significant musculoskeletal symptoms had been documented previously.

Theme: Fracture complications

Options

A	Acute ischaemia	E	Muscle haematoma
B	Compartment syndrome	F	Nerve compression
C	Growth plate disturbance/ damage	G	Sudeck's atrophy – Reflex sympathetic dystrophy
D	Malunion	H	Tendon rupture

For each clinical situation below choose the most likely diagnosis from the list above. Each option may be used once, more than once or not at all).

198. A 15-year-old boy notes a deformity of his right wrist two weeks following the removal of his plaster for a fracture of the distal radius and ulna.

199. A 35-year-old lady presents with severe pain and stiffness of her fingers and hand two weeks following removal of her plaster cast for management of an undisplaced distal radial fracture. She would not allow the doctors to touch her hand, which was noted to be well perfused.

200. A 21-year-old male came to A & E at 3 am complaining of severe agonising pain in his forearm. He would not let anyone move his fingers. He was in a backslab for a displaced fracture of the radius and ulna and been due for admission later that day for an open reduction and internal fixation.

EMQ PRACTICE EXAMINATION – ANSWERS AND EXPLANATIONS

Theme: Colonic disorders

1. **A**

   Carcinoma of the caecum often presents in an insidious way, with a microcytic anaemia, weight loss and sometimes an ache or palpable mass in the right iliac fossa. The large calibre of caecum and liquid consistency of the stool at this point enables these tumours to grow for a long period of time. Unfortunately some of these patients receive several courses of iron tablets before the true diagnosis is reached.

2. **F**

   Irritable bowel syndrome is a diagnosis of exclusion, which typically occurs in younger patients and may be associated with stress or dietary intolerance. Symptoms include constipation, diarrhoea, or both together, associated with cramp-like abdominal pains. Treatment with anti-spasmodic, fibre, or exclusion diets can be tried. Care must be taken to initially rule out any organic pathology.

3. **G**

   Sigmoid volvulus is more common in equatorial countries where the diet is rich in fibre. However, it does occur in temperate countries and usually presents with symptoms of pain and bloating, sometimes as an emergency. A plain abdominal film may demonstrate a large double colonic loop, which is said to resemble a coffee bean.

4. **B**

   Left-sided colonic tumours will more commonly present with an obstructive picture than right-sided tumours. This is due to the more narrow calibre of the colon combined with the more solid consistency of its contents at this point. Typically an annular constricting carcinoma will present with an alteration in bowel habit, change in stool calibre, and finally, frank obstruction. A plain abdominal film may show gross faecal loading proximal to this point, with an absence of bowel gas distally. A contrast enema will usually confirm the diagnosis.

5. **H**

Ulcerative colitis is a disease of unknown aetiology which tends to affect people in the third and fourth decade of life (15% are under the age of 15). It usually presents as a chronic relatively low-grade illness, although 15% of patients may present with fulminant disease. Symptoms include blood-stained diarrhoea, abdominal pain and fever. Extracolonic manifestations include arthritis, iritis, hepatic dysfunction and cutaneous manifestations. The ulceration is superficial, unlike the transmural disease seen in Crohn's colitis.

Theme: Causes of a sore mouth

6.   D

Geographic tongue or erythema migrans is a common autosomal dominant inherited condition that may affect up to 5% of the population. The dorsum of the tongue is affected with migratory areas of depapillation, which may be surrounded by whitish margins. It is often asymptomatic but may give rise to concern when first noticed by the patient or if it leads to rise to soreness whilst eating spicy food.

7.   H

Oral squamous cell carcinoma is the commonest oral malignancy. Its preferred site is the U-shaped area in the floor of the mouth that lies between and includes the lateral border of the tongue and the gum covering the mandible of the lower teeth. It is important to remember that any oral ulcer which has persisted for more than 2 weeks should be biopsied to exclude malignancy. White and red patches in the mouth may be dysplastic or represent carcinoma.

8.   F

Lichen planus is a mucocutaneous disorder that is likely to have an immunological aetiology. The eruption both on the skin and in the mouth tends to be symmetrical. On the skin it tends to start on the flexor surfaces with red and then violaceous pruritic, polygonal, papules which may have white 'Wickham's' striae on their surface. In about 50% of patients the skin lesions resolve within 9 months. Oral involvement tends to be much longer and may be reticular, atrophic or ulcerative. The genitalia may also be involved. Lichen planus, like psoriasis, viral warts and vitiligo, shows Koebner's phenomenon.

9.   E

Iron deficiency may present initially with angular cheilitis and a smooth, red, depapillated, sore tongue. The cause of iron deficiency in this patient may be an occult caecal carcinoma.

10.   J

Poor steroid inhaler technique often results in patients with asthma developing steroid-associated oral candidosis or thrush which may cause an erythematous appearance of the dorsum of the tongue and opposing palate. All patients starting to use such inhalers should have their technique checked, wash their mouth out after inhaler use and if possible use a spacer device to increase delivery of the corticosteroid to the lungs.

Theme: Female urinary incontinence

11. F

Frequency, urgency and dysuria are the classical symptoms of a urinary tract infection for which a MSU is the most appropriate investigation.

12. I

Vaginal bladder repair operations, also called anterior colporrhaphy, are performed to correct a prolapse of the bladder caused by weakness of the pelvic floor muscles or to treat genuine stress incontinence. Patients often present with both conditions. That is the reason for the vaginal route being chosen in the first place. Part of the operation is elevation of the bladder neck to achieve continence. Since the patient is anaesthetised it is the surgeon who has to decide on how tight to pull the stitches around that bladder neck. If they are too loose, the patient will remain incontinent, but if they are too tight, the patient cannot empty her bladder properly. Overflow incontinence results, as described in the scenario. Ultrasound will show an enlarged full bladder.

13. H

Genuine stress incontinence is almost always caused by weakness or damage of the pelvic floor muscles. The main contributing factor is childbirth, and within this a prolonged second stage of labour combined with a big baby. The condition is rarely seen in nulliparous women and can be prevented by elective caesarean section. Consequently exercising the pelvic floor muscles will help the condition and mild cases can even be cured by this measure.

Theme: Petechial rash in a child

14. **E**

Traumatic petechiae or ecchymoses can occur during forceful paroxysms of cough associated with pertussis, foreign body inhalation, etc. The lesions usually occur in the periorbital areas and the lower neck and may be accompanied by subconjunctival haemorrhages. Any other traumatic situation leading to asphyxia needs to be considered.

15. **B**

This is one of the commonest presentations of Henoch Schönlein purpura that causes a generalised vasculitis. The rash is palpable and typically appears in the lower extremity and the buttocks but could involve other areas of the body.

16. **D**

An ill child presenting with a non-blanching purpuric rash has meningococcal septicaemia until proved otherwise and needs rapid treatment with antibiotics and active resuscitation of circulatory volume. This child was in circulatory shock at the time of presentation.

17. **A**

Acute lymphoblastic leukaemia may present with an insidious onset of lethargy and general ill health associated with progressive anaemia and a severe thrombocytopaenia leading to haemorrhages which may be dermal, mucosal or visceral. Clinically there may be lymph node and splenic enlargement.

18. **C**

Idiopathic thrombocytopaenic purpura usually occurs in a healthy child and leads to a sudden onset of a generalised purpuric rash and bruising which is asymmetric. Bleeding can occur from the mucous membranes and severe nosebleeds could occur. Usually there is a history of a viral illness 2–4 weeks previously.

Theme: Acute abdomen

19. **D**

A leaking abdominal aortic aneurysm may mimic many other causes for acute abdomen. The classic triad of a pulsatile mass, severe back pain and profound hypotensive collapse carries a very poor prognosis and these patients frequently do not make it to hospital alive. The clues here are the age, the gender, and the signs of cardiovascular instability.

20. **G**

Non-steroidal anti-inflammatory drugs are widely used, and have a detrimental effect on the kidneys and the gastrointestinal tract. Gas under the diaphragm indicates a perforated viscus and these patients will usually have advanced signs of peritonitis.

21. **H**

The pain of ureteric colic is very severe and will often be described as the worse pain a patient has ever experienced. The characteristic restlessness and inability to find a position that is comfortable is highly suggestive of this condition. A dipstick urine test will usually be positive for blood, and a ureteric calculus will sometimes be seen on the KUB film.

22. **E**

Mesenteric ischaemia occurs in patients who are arteriopaths. Risk factors therefore include an arrhythmia such as atrial fibrillation, advanced age, smoking and diabetes. Postprandial pain and weight loss may denote so-called 'mesenteric angina'. Progression to intestinal gangrene may show as dilated loops of bowel with 'thumbprinting' on a plain abdominal X-ray film, and a blood gas assay may show a metabolic acidosis with profound base deficit. It is a diagnosis of exclusion but the pain the patient experiences may be disproportionately severe to the clinical signs.

23. **A**

The false negative rate for appendicitis is highest in fertile young women and in this group a careful gynaecological history should always be taken and ultrasound scan and even laparoscopy considered. The history for appendicitis is usually brief, 24–48 hours, and will usually be associated with gastrointestinal symptoms such as anorexia, nausea, vomiting or diarrhoea. A longer history, combined with a vaginal discharge is suggestive of pelvic inflammatory disease, but often this diagnosis is only made at the time of removing a normal appendix.

Theme: Otalgia

24. J

Ear canal tumours are rare but the most common type is squamous cell carcinoma. This presents with otorrhoea that may be blood-stained, hearing loss and progressive otalgia. If the middle ear is involved facial paralysis occurs. In addition to local excision, treatment involves mastoidectomy with excision of the parotid gland and temporomandibular joint with postoperative radiotherapy.

25. C

This is a common cause of severe otalgia in children. Eardrum rupture may occur, producing a blood-stained discharge with relief of pain. A swab should be taken for culture and sensitivities. Adults tend to experience loss of balance. Treatment involves bed rest, simple analgesics, nasal decongestants and a broad-spectrum antibiotic to treat streptococci and haemophili. So-called glue ear or otitis media with effusion may affect up to 10% of children (90% of children with cleft palate). These patients should be referred to hospital because of the risk of permanent damage to the middle ear and impaired language development.

26. I

Ramsay Hunt syndrome involves *Herpes zoster* infection of the geniculate ganglion of the facial nerve. Deafness is a complication. Early administration of aciclovir may prevent permanent damage to the facial nerve.

27. E

Referred pain from cervical spondylitis can cause otalgia. Physiotherapy and anti-inflammatory analgesics may be beneficial.

28. K

A carcinoma of the oropharynx may give rise to referred otalgia. Intraoral examination in this patient would show an indurated ulcer affecting the right lateral border of the tongue. Smoking and alcohol consumption are risk factors for oral cancer. Oral pathology ranging from impacted wisdom teeth to carcinoma of the tongue may be causes of referred otalgia. All sites should be visualised and the lymph nodes palpated in patients in whom a cause for otalgia is not immediately obvious.

Theme: Bleeding in pregnancy

29. E

Lower abdominal pain in early pregnancy combined with fainting is highly suspicious of an ectopic pregnancy. Rupture of the ectopic pregnancy may have occurred, with significant intra-abdominal bleeding.

30. H

An 'elderly' multiparous with a significant bleeding at 35 weeks in the absence of pain is highly suspicious of having a placenta praevia. 35 weeks is in fact the classical gestational age for a placenta praevia to bleed. Older age, multiparity, smoking and previous uterine surgery are other recognised risk factors for placenta praevia.

31. F

Insertio velamentosa describes a condition whereby the umbilical vessels are attached to the membranes instead of properly to the placenta. Bleeding from the fetal umbilical cord vessels therefore compromises the fetus and its heart rate will drop. The mother will be largely unaffected, as described in the scenario. Commonly this sort of bleeding is seen in advanced labour when the membranes have ruptured.

32. G

A large-for-dates uterus, exaggerated pregnancy symptoms and heavy vaginal bleeding in the second trimester should raise your suspicion of a molar pregnancy. Pregnancy symptoms are more severe because of the high level of pregnancy hormone and the uterus is large for dates owing to the speed of cell multiplication. The bleeding is heavy because molar tissues are well supplied with blood. Ultrasound would show the famous 'snowstorm picture'. Molar pregnancy can be further divided into partial and complete mole and have a small risk of developing a choriocarcinoma. The other possible cause would be a miscarriage of a multiple pregnancy, but the option is purposely not given.

33. D

This is the classical presentation for a cervical erosion – small bleeding, not fresh, not painful, commonly but not always related to intercourse. Cervical erosions essentially represent an ulcer caused by the fact that endometrial cells migrate to the cervix due to hormone stimulation in pregnancy. When in contact with the acid environment of the vagina, or else 'irritated' by sexual intercourse, they tend to bleed in this particular way. Speculum examination will reveal red areas around the external cervical os. The bleeding is far less than with a placenta praevia, but never the less do not do a pelvic examination before you have excluded this by an ultrasound scan.

Theme: Small stature

34. A

This boy shows signs of early isosexual development and somatic maturation seen in children with late-onset congenital adrenal hyperplasia. As their bone age is far advanced in relation to their chronological age early epiphyseal fusion occurs, leading to a stunted adult height.

35. E

This 6-year-old with an average birth weight and apparent good health has failed to grow within the expected range after an initial 'normal' period. He is far below the expected according to the mid-parental centiles and his height velocity of 2.7 cm for the year is below the 3rd centile indicating growth failure associated with GH deficiency.

36. B

This child has all the features of constitutional delay in growth and puberty with slowing down of his growth indicating a delay of his pubertal growth spurt. He has no evidence of secondary sex characters and has a delayed bone age consistent with the height age. There is usually a family history of delayed puberty, but the ultimate target of achieving the normal adult height is unaffected. For those children who are markedly delayed and are psychologically affected by it, puberty can be initiated with a short course of testosterone

37. D

Genetic or familial short stature usually runs in families, as several close members are affected. The growth velocities of these children remain within normal limits and their bone maturation (bone age) is consistent with the chronological age.

38. C

Her early menarche and the cessation of skeletal growth account for this girl's short stature. Constitutional or idiopathic precocious puberty is more common in girls. Better nutrition and improved general health is said to have lowered the age of menarche, and this is more pronounced among the Asian and Afro-Caribbean populations.

Theme: Low urine output after surgery

39. **D**

Epidural analgesia provides excellent pain control in the postoperative period. Many elderly hypertensive patients require a higher than average mean arterial pressure for renal perfusion and will become oliguric if their blood pressure is lower than usual. This will respond to judicious filling combined with titrating down of the rate of the epidural analgesia.

40. **B**

A small percentage of elderly men will go into acute retention of urine after routine inguinal hernia surgery. This may be caused by a combination of prostatic hypertrophy, combined with the anticholinergic effects of some anaesthetic reversal agents. Pain also contributes. A brief period (24 hours) of catherisation is usually all that is required.

41. **C**

Clot retention is a common problem after TURP and will respond to a bladder washout using strict aseptic technique. Occasionally patients require a return to theatre for further haemostatic diathermy.

42. **A**

Renal failure is occasionally the cause for a low urine output after surgery. Nephrotoxic drugs, hypotension and preoperative impaired renal function are all risk factors.

Theme: Haematological conditions

43. D

B-CLL is the commonest adult leukaemia in the UK, accounting for up to 40% of all leukaemias. The median age of diagnosis is 65–70 years and the male:female ratio is 2:1. It generally follows an indolent course and early on patients are asymptomatic but may have splenomegaly. Lymphadenopathy, anaemia, herpes zoster, bacterial infections, autoimmune haemolysis or thrombocytopenia may cause presentation.

44. H

This clinical scenario is suggestive of multiple myeloma, a tumour of bone marrow plasma cells. Bone pain is the commonest presenting feature and is associated with bone destruction and subsequent hypercalcaemia. Plain radiology may reveal osteoporosis, lytic lesions and evidence of pathological fractures. Renal impairment is common and is usually due to tubular damage caused by Bence Jones protein. Other causes renal impairment in MM includes hypercalcaemia, dehydration, infection, amyloidosis and nonsteroidal inflammatory drugs.

45. A

Acute lymphoblastic leukaemias predominantly affect children and may present with clinical features associated with marrow failure, i.e. anaemia, bleeding and infections. There may also be bone pain, splenomegaly, lymphadenopathy, thymic enlargement and CNS involvement with cranial nerve palsies as in this case. There is a 60% cure rate with chemotherapy.

46. I

Patients with chronic HIV infection are at risk of developing non-Hodgkin's lymphoma

47. E

CML is a clonal disorder of haemopoietic stem cells characterised by the Philadelphia chromosome which is a balanced translocation between chromosomes 9 and 22. It can occur at any age but the median age is 55–60 years with a median survival of 4–5 years. It is a triphasic disease with most patients presenting during the chronic phase which lasts for 2–7 years. In 50% an abrupt transformation into a blast crisis occurs when treatment becomes ineffective. The other 50% undergo an accelerated phase which then proceeds to blast crisis more gradually. If there is a massive neutrophilia there may be associated visual disturbance, priapism or deafness.

Theme: Drugs in gynaecology

48. F

Tranexamic acid is an antifibrinolytic drug, which does not interfere with the menstrual cycle as such, e.g. cycle length or ovulation. It has the ability to reduce menstrual loss by 50% and one in two patients with menorrhagia will benefit from this drug treatment. This makes it very suitable for a woman who is trying to become pregnant.

49. D

One of the non-contraceptive benefits of the oral contraceptive pill (OCP) is regulation of the menstrual cycle. At the age of 17 this young woman is also very likely to require contraception. Other non-contraceptive benefits of the OCP include reduction of menstrual blood loss, improvement of period pains, and reduced likelihood to develop fibroids and a reduced chance to need a hysterectomy. In the long term the OCP reduces the risk of developing endometrial cancer by 50% and of developing ovarian cancer by 40%.

50. C

Primary dysmenorrhoea describes lower abdominal pain before the onset of menstruation, which dissolve once the period has started. The OCP, which is ideal for the treatment of primary dysmenorrhoea, is contraindicated in smokers above the age of 35 owing to an increased risk of a cardiovascular accident. Mefenamic acid is a good alternative without having potentially fatal side-effects like the OCP in these patients.

Theme: Paroxysmal cough in childhood

51. D

The sudden onset of a paroxysmal cough in a previously healthy child in this age group should always bring to mind the possibility of inhalation of a foreign object. In the majority there will be no eyewitness to the incident. The clinical findings will depend on the size and nature of the object inhaled. The common site of involvement is the right lung. In this child the diminished breath sounds and radiological evidence of emphysema of the right lower lobe indicated the site of obstruction.

52. B

Asthma in childhood presents with varying grades of severity. It may present with persistent cough with no history of wheezing, which may occur mainly at night or with exercise. The other common trigger in childhood is viral upper respiratory infections that are treated as 'chest infections' with repeated courses of antibiotics. There will be a history of atopy in the family in most instances.

53. A

A child with a 'persistent cold' is most likely to be suffering from allergic (perennial) rhinitis. The child suffers from nasal obstruction due to mucosal oedema and has a persistent thin mucoid discharge which causes a postnasal drip leading to paroxysmal cough specially at night. The cough could be severe enough to cause vomiting and retching. The constant production of the secretions lead to the noisy breathing and a rattly chest mistakenly treated as asthma.

54. F

Pertussis contracted in early infancy could be life threatening. The early stages may be unrecognised as it may present as an upper respiratory infection but deteriorates rapidly with the onset of paroxysmal cough, cyanotic spells, apnoea and aspiration. Early diagnosis may be facilitated if a contact history is available, but treatment should be started early on suspicion.

Theme: Postoperative fever

55. B

Total parenteral nutrition should only be given through a dedicated feeding line with strict aseptic precautions and close monitoring for line sepsis. Ideally this should be a tunnelled feeding line, but when patients run into unexpected problems the original CVP line placed for monitoring during surgery may be employed for feeding and remain for a longer duration than had been intended. Under these circumstances the risk of sepsis is higher and if it is suspected, the line should be removed immediately, the tip cultured, and a dedicated line placed.

56. A

A fever within the first 48 hours after surgery is usually due to basal atelectasis. Risk factors for this include poor respiration excursion, which may be linked to poor analgesia, an upper abdominal incision such as a Kocher's incision, obesity and poor mobilisation with recumbency.

57. C

Faecal contamination of the peritoneal cavity carries a high morbidity, with a risk of further abscess formation, bacteriaemia and wound infection. Abscess formation should be suspected after the fifth post-operative day and can occur in areas remote from the site of contamination (remember the adage 'pus somewhere, pus nowhere, pus under the diaphragm').

58. E

Appendix perforation is associated with an increased risk of superficial wound infection. This will typically manifest on the fourth or fifth postoperative day and the earliest indication may be a temperature, associated with erythema of the wound, and a thin serosanguineous discharge from the wound edge.

Theme: Causes of oral ulceration

59. H

Herpes zoster of the trigeminal nerve is often preceded by referred pain that may mimic toothache and may result in inappropriate dental extractions. If the ophthalmic division is involved it may result in corneal scarring and visual impairment. Trigeminal nerve shingles has a high association with postherpetic neuralgia. Attacks of shingles are associated with states of reduced immune function such as HIV disease and lymphomas.

60. F

Recurrent oral ulceration affects over one third of the population and most cases are of unknown aetiology. Some cases are associated with haematinic deficiencies or gut malabsorption.

61. A

Behçet's disease is a recurrent multisystem disorder associated with immunologically mediated vasculitis and is characterised by recurrent orogenital ulceration, ocular disease such as anterior uveitis with cutaneous, joint, neurological and vascular involvement. It is a clinical diagnosis but is associated with HLA-B51 and is particularly common in Japan and the Mediterranean countries on the old route along which silk was transported. Other causes of orogenital ulceration include lichen planus, autoimmune vesiculo-bullous disorders such as pemphigus and pemphigoid, erythema multiforme, Reiter's syndrome, herpes simplex virus, HIV, syphilis and gonococcal infection.

62. C

Erythema multiforme is an immunologically mediated mucocutaneous disease that is characterised by numerous target or iris lesions with a central blister affecting the hands and feet. Up to 70% of those affected have painful oral erosions and crusted lips and the genitalia and conjunctivae may also be involved. If severe the disease is termed Stevens-Johnson syndrome. In 50% cases the trigger is not obvious but in the rest herpes simplex virus, HIV, hepatitis B viruses, *Mycoplasma pneumoniae*, various drugs such as penicillin, sulphonamides, barbiturates and malignancy may be implicated.

63. J

Primary syphilis can present in the mouth as described following orogenital contact and more typically affects the tongue. As with genital primary syphilis a small papule breaks down into a large painless chancre and is associated with regional lymphadenopathy. The incubation period is 9–90 days and if left untreated the lesion will heal spontaneously after a period of 1–2 months with subsequent development of the characteristic lesions of secondary syphilis.

Theme: Investigations for suspected malignant disease in gynaecology

64. G

Postmenopausal bleeding may arise from any part of the genital tract and needs to be investigated very promptly and especially cancer of the endometrium excluded. The gold standard investigation is a hysteroscopy combined with a histological specimen from the endometrium. A hysteroscopy is a procedure whereby after dilatation of the cervix a telescope-like instrument is introduced to inspect the uterine cavity. To enhance the view, normal saline or carbon dioxide is used. The advantage over a D&C is that one has a good view and focal lesions such as polyps can be identified and removed. Therefore the combination of the two is ideal. Arguably there is some point in performing a pelvic ultrasound scan to measure the endometrial thickness and exclude adnexal causes. However, this patient is obese, which is a clear limitation for pelvic ultrasound scan and even normal finding would warrant option C. The trilogy of diabetes, obesity and hypertension combined with her age and clinical presentation makes her likely to have an endometrial carcinoma.

65. A

The postmenopausal age of this patient combined with the scan findings are very suspicious of an ovarian malignant process. The fact that she is symptomatic is bad news and indicates advanced disease. A CT scan of the abdomen and pelvis will not alter the fact that she needs a laparotomy over a midline incision but assists in the definition of the extent of the disease and planning of the surgery. Help from urologists and bowel surgeons can be arranged as appropriate. CA 125 is the tumour marker used in epithelial ovarian carcinomas and reflects response to treatment in form of surgery and chemotherapy.

66. E

This 38-year-old patient has not had a smear for 10 years, which is approximately the time span for a normal cervical cell to transform via pre-malignant stages into a cancer cell. Mild, moderate and severe dyskaryosis would have been found over the years in the cytology via smear test and, though not strictly, cervical intraepithelial neoplasia grade 1-3 (CIN I, II and III) found in the histology. Histological specimens of the cervix are taken either by large loop excision of the transformation zone (LLETZ) or cone biopsy. An irregular-looking cervix bleeding easily on touch because of the presence of tumour vessels is highly suspicious of a frank cervical carcinoma. Deep palpation in an outpatient setting may provoke massive haemorrhage and should therefore not been done. Instead, examination under anaesthesia and representative biopsies should be arranged in theatre. The extent of the disease can be evaluated introducing two large Simm's specula in the vagina and biopsies taken. A rectal examination as well as a cystoscopy will give information about infiltration of the neighborhood organs. Depending on this clinical staging but also factors such as coexistent diseases the treatment options are either a radical Wertheim's hysterectomy or radiotherapy.

Theme: Sepsis in childhood

67. H

Children undergoing block chemotherapy for malignancies are susceptible to opportunistic infections due to the marked immunosuppression and accompanying neutropenia that may be induced. Under these circumstances organisms that are normal commensals such as *S. epidermidis* could cause septicaemia especially in those with long-term vascular access via porta caths, picc lines, etc., which may be colonised with the organism.

68. E, G

Chronic infection invariably accelerates the progress of lung disease in cystic fibrosis. The two common organisms associated with this process in CF are *S. aureus* and *P. aeruginosa*. The latter, once ensconced, is difficult to dislodge and requires prolonged and repetitive antibiotic therapy, and is also accompanied by rapid progression of the bronchiectatic process and deterioration of lung function.

69. F

Children with sickle cell disease have impaired reticulo-endothelial or cellular immune function and are prone to develop salmonella infections. The occurrence of infarction in bones, GI tract, etc., makes it easier for the organisms to enter the circulation and provides an ideal environment for localisation.

70. B

Early onset Group B streptococcal infection has a wide spectrum of clinical presentation ranging from asymptomatic bacterial pneumonia to overwhelming septic shock and severe respiratory distress syndrome. Respiratory symptoms are predominant including cyanosis, apnoea, grunting and tachypnoea and variable X-ray findings. The early onset disease is due to serotypes present in the colonised mother.

71. G

This child's symptoms, signs and the markedly elevated inflammatory markers are compatible with an osteomyelitis of the right tibia, though it is too early to expect any radiological changes. A bone scan could be diagnostic in the early stages. The commonest organism responsible in over 90% of the cases is *Staphylococcus aureus*.

72. **A**

This child presented with symptoms and signs of a septicaemia, subsequently shown to be associated with a urinary tract infection, i.e. acute pyelonephritis. The commonest organism associated with urinary tract infection in up to 90% of girls is *E. coli.*

Theme : Thyroid malignancies

73. C

Lymphoma of the thyroid gland is often forgotten as a cause of thyroid swelling. Its presentation in some ways resembles anaplastic carcinoma of the thyroid gland, but it is even rarer (4% versus 13%) and has a gender bias towards female patients.

74 and 76 D

Medullary carcinoma of the thyroid gland arises from the parafollicular C cells which are neural crest cell derivatives. These tumours produce high levels of serum calcitonin, which provides a valuable tumour marker, the level falling after surgical resection. Medullary carcinoma can occur as part of the multiple endocrine neoplasias (MEN type 2A), when it is associated with adrenal pheochromocytoma and hyperparathyroidism.

75. B

Follicular carcinoma accounts for approximately 20% of thyroid cancers and typically occurs in the fifth decade of life. 50% of them are minimally invasive and associated with an excellent prognosis. 50% of patients with invasive follicular carcinoma develop local recurrence or secondary spread (typically bone or lung) and have a mean survival time of 6 years after surgery.

Theme: Orofacial manifestations of systemic disease

77. J

Nifedipine is well recognised as a cause of gingival hyperplasia when used in patients with poor oral hygiene. Treatment involves improving plaque control and may require gingivectomy. Cyclosporin and phenytoin are other recognised causes of gingival hyperplasia.

78. D

C1 esterase deficiency or hereditary angioedema presents with recurrent attacks of oedema affecting the subcutaneous tissues and submucosa. It is inherited in an autosomal dominant fashion and individuals affected have defective production of C1 esterase inhibitor by one of the two genes on chromosome 11 involved in its production. Complement profiles show low levels of C2 and C4. The face, tongue and upper airway may be involved, giving rise to respiratory embarrassment. Bowel wall involvement may result in severe abdominal pain. Episodes last for up to 4 days and may occur sporadically or triggered by psychological stress or physical trauma. Individuals may be affected from childhood. Anabolic steroids or androgens are effective in reducing the frequency and severity of attacks. Epinephrine, corticosteroids and antihistamines are of no benefit. Rarely acquired C1 esterase inhibitor deficiency may occur in autoimmune diseases such as SLE or haematological malignant diseases.

79. L

Intermittent parotid swelling is a feature of Sjögren's syndrome. This relatively common autoimmune disease causes oral and ocular dryness and has a strong female predilection. The disease may occur in association with another autoimmune connective disease such as SLE or rheumatoid arthritis, when it is described as secondary Sjögren's syndrome.

80. C

This is a classical presentation of bulimia nervosa. The bilateral parotid swelling occurs following working hypertrophy of the salivary glands and the calluses occur secondary to the use of the fingers to stimulate vomiting. Examination of the palatal surfaces of the upper teeth may also show erosion from the acidic vomit.

81. **H**

    These oral lesions represent oral hairy leukoplakia and are caused by infection of the oral epithelial cells by Epstein-Barr virus. In addition to being found in patients with advanced HIV disease they may also be seen in other immunosuppressed patients such as those with renal transplants and even those who use corticosteroid inhalers for asthma.

Theme: Management of labour

82. G

An 'empty' pelvis refers to the fact that the presenting part has not engaged to the pelvic outlet. Vaginally there is only cervix palpable, which may be to some degree dilated, the bony and soft tissues of the maternal pelvis and above the ischial spines an empty space. In a cephalic presentation the fetal head fills out this space. However, in the given scenario malpresentation of the fetus has to be ruled out by ultrasound. Commonly there is a breech presentation, which tends to engage later in labour, but transverse lie of the fetus is also a possibility.

83. B

Meconium is found in about 40% of term pregnancies and in most cases represents simply maturity of the fetus. However, it is a well-known fact that oxygen deprivation of the fetus can also go along with release of meconium. Therefore additional tests have to be performed. Cardiotocography (CTG) is the traditional way to monitor fetal well-being. Abnormal findings there in conjunction with meconium necessitates delivery since there is a high risk of oxygen deprivation of the fetus. In a primiparous woman with the cervix only 2 cm dilated an emergency caesarean section has to be performed. A fetal blood sample would be technically very difficult to do. Also given the average time of labour is 12 hours in a primiparous woman and the fetus is very likely compromised, an emergency caesarean is justified.

84. E

Malposition of the fetal head is one of the most common causes for failure to progress in labour. This woman has been 4 hours in the second stage and deserves to be delivered. The fetal head should be almost visible and instrumental vaginal delivery, by either forceps or ventouse, has a good chance of success.

85. C

Variable deceleration describes a mixture or early and late deceleration. Compression of the umbilical cord is the common cause for this CTG finding. However, it is advisable to perform a definite test, which is a fetal blood sample from the baby's scalp, and measure the pH. In advanced labour, when the cervix is sufficiently dilated, there is good and easy access to the baby's head via an amnioscope.

86. **A**

Any circumstances other than the norm require continuous CTG monitoring in labour to ensure timely intervention as necessary. A small-for-dates fetus is no exception.

Theme: *Chronic diarrhoea in infancy and childhood*

87. G

Chronic inflammatory bowel disease in the form of ulcerative colitis presents in adolescence and usually manifests constitutional symptoms and signs at the time of diagnosis. Though extra-intestinal manifestations are uncommon when compared to adult disease, their presence will help in earlier diagnosis. These include arthritis, erythema nodosum, rarely hepatitis and pyoderma gangrenosum.

88. F

This is non-specific diarrhoea with no evidence of malabsorption or other inflammatory cause where the affected child is healthy, developing and thriving normally. There is no associated weight loss, dehydration or electrolyte imbalance and it is considered to be due to a shorter intestinal transit time.

89. A

Any infant with chronic respiratory symptoms and chronic diarrhoea and failure to thrive needs to be screened for cystic fibrosis. The child may present with one or the other symptom predominating.

90. C

Typically, in gluten enteropathy symptoms develop in the latter part of the first year after weaning to solids and hence to gluten-containing food. The clinical manifestations are variable, from severe malabsorption – the child with wasting, anaemia and lack of growth – to apparent normal health. Screening tests such as IgA anti endomysial and anti reticulin antibodies are helpful in the diagnosis, as they are highly specific.

91. D

An infant with a combination of symptoms of constipation and diarrhoea associated with abdominal distension and who had delayed passage of meconium is most likely to have Hirschsprung disease. The symptoms can vary from complete neonatal intestinal obstruction to profuse diarrhoea due to an enterocolitis. Diagnosis is by rectal biopsy.

Theme: Biliary tract

92. C

Sphincterotomy and extraction of biliary tract stones plus stenting if necessary are common manoeuvres during ERCP.

93. D

A persistently elevated amylase several days or weeks after an attack of pancreatitis may be a clue to the formation of a pancreatic pseudocyst.

94. E

A combination of elevated alkaline phosphatase and bilirubin with normal transamylase levels is indicative of obstruction of the common bile duct. Gallstones are frequently responsible for this.

95. F

Prognostic indicators for acute pancreatitis include age over 55, raised white count, blood glucose, LDH, AST, urea, a fall in haematocrit and calcium, and blood gas derangement. Surprisingly amylase is not of prognostic value, but is only useful to make the initial diagnosis.

96. C

Endoscopic Retrograde Cholangio Pancreatography (ERCP) can cause pancreatitis. This is thought to be due to pancreatic ductal over distension.

Theme: Facial appearance

97. K

Seborrhoeic dermatitis may be associated with overgrowth of *Pityrosporum ovale*, commensal yeast, and can be severe in patients with HIV disease. The eruption often affects sebaceous areas of the skin. Scalp and facial involvement is a common presentation in young men.

98. L

Skin signs are present in approximately three-quarters of patients with systemic lupus erythematosus (SLE). They may consist of a facial butterfly rash, photosensitivity, round or oval discoid lesions, diffuse alopecia and vasculitis and occur in association with other organ involvement as well as immunological abnormalities such as circulating antinuclear autoantibodies. In discoid lupus erythematosus (DLE) involvement is confined to the skin, with scaly round or oval red plaques appearing on the face, scalp or hands. Multisystem involvement is not a feature although 5% may subsequently develop into SLE. Women are significantly more frequently affected in SLE (female:male ratio of up to 9:1) but in DLE the ratio drops to 2:1.

99. J

Sarcoidosis may affect the skin in up to one-third of cases. The skin changes are variable. On the face there may be violaceous or brownish red papules and the term lupus pernio may be used to describe dusky-red infiltrated plaques on the nose. There may be associated erythema nodosum usually in white women with bilateral hilar lymphadenopathy. Chest examination may be normal. Treatment involves intralesional steroids or if there is significant internal organ involvement oral steroids or methotrexate may be used. Lupus vulgaris describes the cutaneous form of tuberculosis and occurs in people with a moderate to high degree of immunity. The soft reddish-brown plaques commonly occur on facial or neck skin and tend to be associated with scarring.

100. H

Peutz-Jeghers syndrome is a rare autosomal dominant condition in which affected patients have lentigenes around and in the mouth and on the fingers as well as small and large bowel polyps. The bowel polyps can cause intestinal obstruction and rarely undergo malignant change.

101. A

Rosacea is a chronic inflammatory facial skin disorder of unknown aetiology. It is characteristically erythematous and pustular. It is commonest in middle age and in men may be associated with rhinophyma, that is to say hyperplasia of the connective tissue and sebaceous glands of the nose. Topical metronidazole gel may be helpful.

Theme: Causes for amenorrhoea

102. C

Normal secondary characteristics, which include breast development and typical female hair distribution in the axilla and the pubic area, make endocrine and chromosomal causes for amenorrhoea very unlikely. The fact that she has cyclical abdominal pain pretty much implies an outflow obstruction of which an imperforate hymen is the commonest form. This is not associated with abnormalities of the renal tract.

103. A

Normal secondary characteristics and normal endocrine results leaves you to explore anatomical causes again. The progesterone challenge test is performed by giving medroxyprogesterone acetate 5 mg TDS for 5 days. If positive, vaginal bleeding will occur reflecting the presence of a functioning endometrium and an intact outflow tract. If negative, one or the other of these is not working. Since no other options are given and the patient is asymptomatic, absence of the uterus is the most likely cause.

104. E

Sheehan's syndrome is a rare, but classic complication of massive postpartum haemorrhage. Necrosis of the anterior lobe of the hypophysis is the anatomical correlate, causing failure of all the hormones produces there. Secondary amenorrhoea is therefore only one feature.

105. F

Short stature associated with a variety of other findings is a classic feature of Turner syndrome or XO-karyotype. Secondary sexually characteristics are absent or maldeveloped owing to oestrogen deficiency. For the same reason these patients are amenorrhoeic.

Theme: Fits and faints in children

106. G

Simple syncope results from transient fall in blood pressure due to vasovagal stimulation (dysautonomia syncope) by a variety of stimuli such as pain, fear and standing for a long time, especially in a warm environment. There is a prodrome of dizziness, nausea, buzzing sensation in ears, pallor, sweating and loss of tone followed by loss of consciousness. The EEG does not show epileptic discharges during the episode.

107. A

This child has typical features of benign paroxysmal vertigo. There is no loss of consciousness, the main feature being transient ataxia. During an attack horizontal nystagmus may be noted. There is increased tendency to suffer from motion sickness.

108. B

This child has typical breath-holding attacks that are precipitated by her being upset and angry. Expiration and apnoea, leading to cyanosis and loss of consciousness, follow the initial cry. The child is bradycardic and may exhibit a few jerky movements.

109. C

This child has complex partial seizures. There appears to be an aura and some lateralisation at the onset of the seizure that subsequently becomes generalised.

110. E

Reflex anoxic syncope first appears around 1 year of age and is precipitated by sudden pain or fright. The child stops breathing and rapidly loses consciousness, becoming hypotonic and pale. There may be a tonic seizure. There is marked bradycardia or a short period of asystole. Recovery is spontaneous and rarely requires intervention.

Theme: Hair loss

111. F

Both lichen planus and lupus erythematosus can lead to a scarring alopecia in addition to other cutaneous involvement. The lesions may respond to topical or intralesional corticosteroids or systemic therapy.

112. A

Alopecia areata is a common autoimmune condition that may start in the second or third decade. It presents with sharply defined areas of alopecia that are non-erythematous. The eyebrows and beard may also be involved. The nails may show pitting. Classically so-called exclamation-mark hairs are found in affected areas that taper towards the scalp.

113. K

Childbirth, high fevers, illness and other stresses may result in all the growth cycles of the scalp hair follicles becoming synchronized into the telogen resting mode resulting in uniform hair shedding occurring 3 months later.

114. B

So-called male pattern or androgenetic hair loss may also occur in women, particularly after the menopause. They may demonstrate the typical male pattern hair loss with bitemporal recession and a bald crown or diffuse thinning of the hair. Minoxidil may stimulate some regrowth in one-third of patients. Androgen-secreting tumours in women may present with virilization and male pattern baldness.

115. D

Both underactivity and overactivity of the thyroid gland can result in diffuse hair loss, as can hypopituitarism and hypoadrenalism.

Theme: Investigations in pregnancy

116. F

The Kleihauer test demonstrates fetal red cells in the maternal blood circulation and according to the test result Anti-D immunoglobulin injection is given to the mother to destroy rhesus positive fetal cells thereby preventing the mother from forming Anti-D antibodies. The Kleihauer test is used whenever a rhesus negative woman has significant bleeding in pregnancy. As a precaution, all of these women are assumed to carry a rhesus positive fetus since rhesus iso-immunisation can have devastating effects on future pregnancies.

117. C

Thirty- five weeks is the typical gestational age for the development of cholestasis in pregnancy. This presents mainly with itching, only very rarely with jaundice and is associated with an increased risk of perinatal morbidity and mortality. Classically, the liver function parameters are only mildly elevated but the bile acids are significantly increased. Antihistamines and cholestyramine, which is a bile acid chelating agent, may be used to treat the itching. Close fetal surveillance and delivery at 38 weeks are advised for the above reasons.

118. A

A diastolic blood pressure of more than 90 combined with proteinuria warrants further investigation. Pre-eclampsia is a very likely diagnosis here. The urine dipstick is a qualitative test; it is designed to confirm the presence or absence of e.g. protein in a sample. Once positive, the quantitative test in form of a 24 hour urine collection has to be used to exactly measure the protein excretion. 300 ml or less per 24 hours is normal in pregnancy; readings above this have to be appraised in the context of the clinical picture.

119. D

The symphysial-fundal height roughly corresponds to the gestational age, e.g. 35 cm roughly equals 35 weeks of gestation. Intrauterine growth restriction is a condition whereby the fetus fails to achieve its growth potential. Causes for this are either maternal, e.g. smoking or hypertension, fetal, e.g. chromosomal or structural abnormalities, or placental. Close surveillance of the fetus is indicated and ultrasound is one of the standard investigations. Doppler ultrasound of the umbilical artery gives information on the quality on blood supply of the fetus and according to these results delivery can be planned.

120. B

The triple test is a screening test for Down's syndrome offered to all women in the UK. The blood sample is taken between 15 and 17 weeks of pregnancy and levels of beta-HCG, alpha-fetoprotein and oestriol are measured and by taking the age of the mother into account, a risk is calculated for the fetus to be affected by Down's syndrome. Amniocentesis is the definitive test offered to women at increased risk. Under ultrasound guidance a thin needle is inserted through the mother's abdomen and a small amount of the amniotic fluid around the baby withdrawn.

Theme: *Investigation of neuromuscular disease*

121. A

The most likely cause for the seizures in this small-for-dates baby is hypoglycaemia. They are very susceptible, due to the low glycogen stores and inadequate intake in the first few days until the establishment of feeding. It is vital to monitor the blood glucose regularly and to give sufficient either via supplementary feeds or intravenously until stabilised.

122. C

This child has delayed motor development and shows clinical features of proximal muscle weakness using the Gower's manoeuvre to stand up. Duchenne muscular dystrophy needs to be eliminated and initially a CPK level will be needed.

123. G

This child has vomiting, possibly headaches which make him miserable, change in behaviour, ataxia and possibly early papillo-edema, all indicative of increased intracranial pressure due to a space-occupying lesion. An urgent MRI is indicated, as it is 100% sensitive in the diagnosis of brain tumours.

124. F

This baby has recurrent flexor spasms associated with some evidence of developmental arrest. The most likely diagnosis is infantile spasms. An urgent EEG will confirm this with a typical hypsarrhythmia pattern.

125. B

This baby has features suggestive of Down's syndrome though not typical. Excessive hypotonia with feeding problems and a few stigmata of Down's necessitates a chromosomal analysis for a definitive diagnosis to be made early.

126. E

The bradycardia and associated cardiac enlargement in a previously healthy child detracts from a diagnosis of complex cardiac disease. This child needs an ECG to determine the nature of the bradycardia, which most likely is a complete heart block of congenital origin.

Theme: Causes of dysphagia

127. J

Gastro-oesophageal reflux disease (GORD) is associated with smoking, high alcohol intake, hiatus hernia, pregnancy, obesity, systemic sclerosis and tight clothes. Gastric acid is permitted to enter the oesophagus through the incompetent lower oesophageal sphincter. This results in oesophageal inflammation, which if extensive may result in dysphagia and eventually oesophageal stricture or Barrett's oesophagus. Patients may complain of heartburn, an acid taste in the mouth (acid brash), excessive salivation (waterbrash), difficulty in swallowing, and nocturnal asthma.

128. A

Oesophageal achalasia involves failure of relaxation of the circular muscles at the lower end of the oesophagus associated with loss of the myenteric plexus of nerves in this region. Oesophageal dilatation occurs above the area of achalasia. The condition tends to present between the ages of 30–40 years and is slightly more common in women. Dysphagia gradually progresses over years. In addition to regurgitation of partially digested food, halitosis and foul eruptation patients may aspirate on lying flat (hence the coughing) and so are susceptible to aspiration pneumonia. The diagnosis may be obvious on a chest radiograph with a wide mediastinum and a shadow behind the heart with a fluid level. Further confirmation of the diagnosis can be obtained with a barium swallow or oesophagoduodenoscopy. Treatment of severe achalasia is usually surgical (Heller's operation) but mild achalasia may respond to nitrates and anticholinergic medication.

129. I

Plummer-Vinson syndrome or Paterson-Brown-Kelly syndrome consists of iron deficiency anaemia, glossitis, angular cheilitis and dysphagia due to a postcricoid oesophageal web. A friable web lies across the anterior oesophageal lumen and may be seen on endoscopy and a barium meal. It is caused by epithelial hyperplasia and hyperkeratosis of the oesophageal mucosa. The condition is premalignant and should be biopsied. The iron deficiency anaemia should be investigated and treated appropriately.

130. H

The development of a pharyngeal pouch is often preceded by a history suggestive of reflux oesophagitis or hiatus hernia. It has been hypothesised that oesophageal hypertrophy occurs in an attempt to prevent acid reflux and that this causes a relative obstruction at the level of cricopharyngeus muscle with the resultant pressure causing protrusion of a mucosal pouch at the level of Killian's dehiscence between thyreopharyngeus and cricopharyngeus. This pouch is usually easily demonstrated in the upper neck on a barium swallow. Again patients are prone to aspiration of semi-digested food which leads to episodes of coughing and aspiration pneumonia. Management is surgical with excision of the pouch.

131. E

The description of the clinical findings suggests that this patient has significant mitral stenosis. The associated large left atrium may favour atrial fibrillation with palpitations and pressure on the oesophagus may result in dysphagia. Radiological features in mitral stenosis associated with enlargement of the left atrium include a double cardiac silhouette, straightening of the left border of the heart and a horizontal left bronchus.

Theme: Health benefits from contraceptives

132. B

It is one of the known non-contraceptive benefits of the combined oral contraceptive pill that in users the risk of endometrial cancer is reduced by 50%. Ovarian cancer risk is reduced by 40%.

133. A

Sexually transmitted diseases are reduced by barrier methods, which is common sense.

134. D

Depo-Provera injections provide 150 mg of medroxyprogesterone acetate at once by intramuscular. injection and need to be repeated every 3 months to provide reliable contraception. One of the good indications is to give it as a postpartum contraceptive to a breastfeeding mother. It improves the quality of the breast milk because of the high dose of progestogens, which have a synergistic effect on milk production.

135. B

Primary dysmenorrhoea is a reflection of ovulatory menstrual cycles. Inhibition of ovulation therefore has a beneficial effect. The combined oral contraceptive pill is a classical example.

136. E

The Mirena coil is one of the newer intrauterine contraceptive devices, which releases minimal doses of levonorgestrel every day and is effective for 5 years. The foreign body in the form of the coil acts as a contraceptive and the small doses of levonorgestrel will slim down the endometrium thereby reducing menstrual loss over a time span of 4–9 months. The combined oral contraceptive pill contains synthetic forms of oestrogen, mainly ethinyloestradiol, and this poses an increased risk of cardiovascular accidents to smokers over 35 years of age. It is therefore contraindicated.

Theme: Investigation of neonatal jaundice

137. G

This baby has clinical evidence of a significant infection. The clinical features, accompanied by elevated WBC and neutrophil counts, CRP, and the metabolic acidosis indicate a bacterial sepsis that will exaggerate physiological jaundice. Under the circumstances blood, urine and CSF cultures are mandatory and antibiotics need to be started empirically.

138. C

This baby's rapidly increasing jaundice is due to severe haemolysis as indicated by the low haemoglobin and high indirect bilirubin. Unlike the situation in blood group incompatibility between mother and infant, here the haemolysis has occurred later. Considering the parental ethnicity the most likely cause is a membrane defect of the red cells such as G6PD deficiency. It is vital to get information regarding maternal ingestion of food or medication that may pass through breast milk into the baby.

139. D

This ill baby has hypoglycaemia leading to seizures associated with jaundice, hepatomegaly, presence of reducing substances in urine (non-glucose) and elevated liver enzymes that is typically present in galactosaemia.

140. F

This baby shows the presence of hepatitis with elevated direct and indirect bilirubin and liver enzymes. The cause of the hepatitis can be surmised to be congenital syphilis by mother's lack of antenatal care and therefore missing routine serological investigations and the baby's clinical features of snuffles with periostitis of the humerus noted on the chest X-ray. This was confirmed by serology.

Theme: Pruritus

141. E

Lichen planus is a chronic mucocutaneous dermatosis of unknown aetiology which in the mouth can give rise to chronic areas of white striae, plaques and erosions. It may be sore, particularly when spicy foods are eaten. On the skin lesions generally consist of violaceous polygonal papules which are intensely itchy. They are classically found on the skin of the flexor surfaces of the wrist and shins. Oral and skin lesions may respond to topical corticosteroid preparations. Nail involvement results in pitting, ridging and loss in severe cases. Scalp involvement may lead to alopecia.

142. B

Dermatitis herpetiformis is an uncommon symmetrical vesiculo-bullous disorder that typically affects the extensor surfaces. It usually presents in the third or fourth decade and is twice as common in men as in women. The blisters are rarely found intact, usually being excoriated. Most patients have associated jejunal villus atrophy but symptoms of gastrointestinal disturbance and malabsorption are unusual. Antiendomysial antibodies are present and skin biopsy shows Ig deposits along the dermal papillae. A gluten-free diet is the treatment of choice. Dapsone will also control the eruption and may be given until the diet has had time to work.

143. I

Polycythaemia rubra vera may present with neurological signs related to hyperviscosity such as cerebral ischaemic events or visual disturbances, angina, Raynaud's syndrome, and itch which is typically worse after a hot bath. Gout may also occur owing to increased red cell turnover. There may also be associated bruising. Splenomegaly may occur. Treatment involves venesection or the use of hydroxyurea to keep the packed cell volume below 50%. Prognosis is variable.

144. G

Hodgkin's lymphoma often presents with enlarged painless lymph nodes which due to their size may cause pressure effects. Approximately 25% have systemic features such as weight loss, fever, night sweats, pruritus and lethargy. The Ann Arbor staging subdivides each stage into (A) non-systemic features other than pruritus and (B) presence of weight loss >10% in the last 6 months, unexplained fever > 38°C or night sweats and signifies more extensive disease and worse prognosis.

145. D

Iron deficiency may result in koilonychia, spoon-shaped nails that are brittle, atrophic glossitis with associated inflammation at the angles of the mouth, so-called angular cheilitis, pruritus and postcricoid webs (Plummer-Vinson syndrome). In this age group iron deficiency may be result of a poor diet but may also reflect underlying occult gastrointestinal blood loss, for example from a colonic malignancy.

Theme: Convulsion in pregnancy

146. A

Age, hypertension, heavy cigarette smoking combined with pregnancy make an atherosclerotic cause for convulsion very likely, and cerebral infarction is the one to choose from the possible answers.

147. D

This patient's young age without a previous medical history and a sudden rise of her blood pressure implies on its own a pregnancy-related cause for convulsion. Most likely she has an eclamptic fit.

148. C

There is a history of drug abuse and since gastric emptying is delayed due to the progesterone effect on the gastrointestinal tract, insufficient drug levels in the plasma may be the cause for convulsion.

149. B

Repeated pregnancy loss and deep vein thrombosis is altogether very suspicious of a clotting disorder, either an isolated factor deficiency, e.g. protein C or S deficiency, mutation of factor Leiden V or a so-called anti-phospholipid antibody syndrome. Therefore a thrombotic event would be the likely option to choose.

Theme: Heart disease in childhood

150. E

Delayed closure of the ductus in preterm babies may cause deterioration following earlier recovery from RDS. This is an important differential diagnosis that needs to be considered in babies who are difficult to wean off ventilators or remain oxygen dependent for a longer period. This baby has the typical haemodynamic features of PDA.

151. C

This child demonstrates all the clinical features of heart failure. The onset of the heart failure following a previous infection associated with gross cardiac enlargement is indicative of a dilated cardiomyopathy following a myocarditis. Assessment of the left ventricular function by echocardiography is a vital investigation that may help in prognostication and planning treatment.

152. F

This baby has Fallot's tetralogy and shows typical clinical findings. The diagnosis is easily confirmed by echocardiography. The progression of cyanosis is variable and depends on the severity of the pulmonary stenosis: the more severe the PS, the earlier in infancy the appearance of cyanosis. Measurement of the O_2 saturation will help to identify these children before onset of cyanosis.

153. A

Clinical features are suggestive of left ventricular outflow obstruction. In older children effort induced syncope or chest pain could be the presenting feature. Echocardiography is diagnostic as left ventricular function and the gradient across the narrowed valve can be accurately assessed.

154. B

This baby too presents in cardiac failure. The clinical features are of a large left to right shunt due to a VSD but the superior QRS axis is a feature of a complete AV septal defect. The diagnosis is easily confirmed by echocardiography. In addition to the rapid control of the failure early surgery is indicated, as there is a higher risk of developing pulmonary hypertension.

Theme: Findings on physical examination

155. I

Myasthenia gravis is a relatively rare autoimmune disorder in which antibodies are produced to the acetylcholine receptors of the neuromuscular junction. Although any muscle may be affected, most patients have ptosis and many have ophthalmoplegia, dysarthria and dysphagia. The pupil is not affected. In comparison, LEMS may be a paraneoplastic disorder associated with small cell carcinoma of the lung or less commonly breast and ovarian carcinoma. It involves autoantibodies to voltage-gated calcium channels in the muscle membrane. In contrast to myasthenia gravis, in LEMS ophthalmoplegia and ptosis are not features; although reflexes are absent or reduced initially they improve with exercise and the proximal limb muscles and trunk are affected

156. C

A number of the clinical features of chronic liver disease are described in this patient whose liver disease may be secondary to hepatitis B or C infection due to the use of intravenous drugs. Other associated features include Dupuytren's contracture, spider naevi, testicular atrophy and parotid enlargement. Cirrhosis and excessive alcohol consumption are two of a number of recognized associations with gynaecomastia which are due to decreased androgen/oestrogen ratio in men.

157. E

Holmes-Adie pupil is a benign condition involving moderate usually unilateral pupillary dilatation that typically affects women. The affected dilated pupil is poorly reactive to light and is slowly reactive to accommodation. When it is associated with reduced or absent knee and ankle reflexes it is known as the Holmes-Adie syndrome.

158. J

This is a classical presentation of a pericardial effusion. However, these symptoms may be absent. Significant effusions may lead to muffled heart sounds, absent apical impulse, pulsus alternans, pulsus paradoxus with small ECG complexes and cardiac enlargement on chest X-ray.

159. B

Bronchial carcinoma is a recognized cause of finger clubbing. Other associated respiratory causes include chronic lung suppuration (lung abscess, empyema, bronchiectasis, cystic fibrosis), fibrosing alveolitis and mesothelioma.

Theme: Diagnosis in gynaecology

160. F

This is the very typical clinical picture of a ruptured ovarian cyst.

161. D

Lower abdominal pain, deep dyspareunia, subfertility and also secondary dysmenorrhoea are the clinical features of endometriosis. The comment about the stable relationship implies that pelvic inflammatory disease should not be your first choice of answer.

162. C

This patient is of premenopausal age noticing a swelling of the abdominal circumference together with weight loss and constipation. One has to think of a malignant, probably already advanced, ovarian tumour.

163. B

Irritable bowel syndrome is the commonest cause for lower abdominal pain in young women. Very typically, findings at laparoscopy are negative and so are the swab results, directing you again away from pelvic inflammatory disease. In fact 60% of diagnostic laparoscopies are negative, which is very important to remember when counselling these patients preoperatively.

Theme: Drug treatment in childhood

164. A

Co-trimoxazole is the drug of choice in the treatment of *Pneumocystis carinii* pneumonia and is usually given as a 2-week course.

165. J

This infant has tuberous sclerosis. Vigabatrin is considered to be a first choice anticonvulsant in the treatment of seizures in TS.

166. D

This baby has clinical features of a VSD with a large left to right shunt leading to cardiac failure that has not responded to diuretics. An ACE inhibitor such as enalapril will improve the cardiac function by reducing the 'pre' and 'after' load.

167. G

Rifampicin is given to the contacts of meningococcal patients.

168. E

This baby has a symptomatic persistent PDA which has not responded to fluid restriction. The drug of choice is indomethacin given orally or intravenously as a 3 or 6 day course. Careful monitoring of renal function and coagulation is required. It is contra-indicated in the presence of sepsis or where a duct-dependent circulation needs to be maintained.

169. J

This child has typical clinical and EEG features of infantile spasms. Previously treated with ACTH or prednisolone, now the preferred choice is vigabatrin.

170. I

This organism may respond to vancomycin given intravenously. It is important to be aware of its nephrotoxic and ototoxic potential and monitor the patient carefully.

Theme: Autoantibodies

171. F

Neonates born to mothers with anti-Ro autoantibodies develop neonatal lupus erythematosus with permanent heart block owing to antigenic cross-reactivity with the antigens in cardiac conducting tissue. The IgG autoantibodies cross the placenta and are passively acquired. Affected infants require permanent pacing but other associated features such as rash, leukopenia and hepatitis are temporary and resolve by 6 months.

172. I

This describes drug-induced lupus which may be associated with slow acetylator status and HLA DR4. Drugs such as isoniazid, hydralazine, procainamide, chlorpromazine and anticonvulsants may precipitate it. Cutaneous and pulmonary signs predominate over renal and CNS signs. It remits on stopping the drug. ANA are positive but ds-DNA is negative.

173. A

The antimichondrial M2 antibody is found in a high percentage of patients with primary biliary cirrhosis

174. H

Anticentromere autoantibodies are associated with limited cutaneous systemic sclerosis formerly described as CREST syndrome.

175. J

This patient has rheumatoid arthritis with rheumatoid nodules which are always associated with rheumatoid factor and a more severe arthritis.

Theme: Adverse drug effects

176. F

A large number of drugs including digoxin, spironolactone, stilboestrol, cimetidine, ketoconazole, metronidazole, cyproterone acetate and griseofulvin have been associated with gynaecomastia. Gynaecomastia involves increased breast glandular material and is unrelated to galactorrhoea.

177. G

Methotrexate may cause a severe mucositis as well as myelosuppression if used without folinic acid rescue.

178. J

Retinoids are used by dermatologists for the treatment of severe psoriasis and acne. They are teratogenic and have a large range side-effects including alopecia, hypertriglyceridaemia, hepatitis, altered mood, hepatitis and benign intracranial hypertension. Mucous membrane dryness may lead to intolerance of contact lenses.

179. A

Phenothiazines, mepacrine, chloroquine, busulphan, clofazimine and minocycline may all cause cutaneous pigmentation. Bleomycin may cause diffuse pigmentation that is often flexural. Amiodarone causes blue-grey pigmentation of sun-exposed areas.

180. E

Cyclosporin may also cause dose-dependent nephrotoxicity, hypertension, potassium and fluid retention, liver dysfunction, and gingival hyperplasia in addition to hirsutism. In the first week of therapy it may also cause the sensation of burning hands and feet.

Theme: Arterial pulses

181. D

With a collapsing pulse the pulse pressure is greater than diastolic pressure. A collapsing pulse may also be found in patients with patent ductus arteriosus or an arterio-venous fistula.

182. F

A paradoxical pulse also occurs in left ventricular compression, constrictive pericarditis or severe asthma.

183. B

Pulsus alterans or alternating pulses describes a pulse with a regular rhythm but with alternating beats which are weak and then strong. It is found in patients with severe heart failure and suggests a poor prognosis i.e. fleeting prolonged recovery of the failing heart muscles.

184. G

Pulse which is slow rising and plateaus is found in moderate or severe aortic stenosis.

185. A

This idiopathic arteritis typically affects women between the ages of 20–40 years. It results in narrowing of major arteries such as the renal, carotid, innominate and subclavian as well as the adjacent aorta. Cardiovascular examination may demonstrate absent pulses, aortic regurgitation, systolic murmurs above and below the clavicle and hypertension if the renal arteries are involved. Other causes of an absent radial pulse includes trauma, dissection of the aorta with subclavian involvement, peripheral arterial embolus and post catheterisation iatrogenic damage.

Theme: Psychiatric presentations

186. B

A number of the clinical features of mania are described. For the ICD-10 diagnostic criteria to be fulfilled there should be a history of at least two episodes of mood disturbance at least one of which should have been mania or hypomania. On average the age of onset is in the mid-twenties. The main differential diagnoses are schizophrenia and organic psychoses. Cyclothymia describes a persisting instability of mood with multiple episodes of mild elation and depression. Again it usually presents early in adult life.

187. I

Seasonal affective disorder involves the onset of depression at a particular season. There may be associated carbohydrate craving, hypersomnia and weight gain.

188. J

Somatization disorder is a type of somatoform disorder. Other examples include hypochondriacal disorder and persistent somatoform pain disorder. All affected patients present repeatedly with physical symptoms and are not reassured by normal clinical examinations and negative investigation results.

Theme: Red eyes

189. C

This describes the typical presentation of anterior uveitis and the brief history is suggestive of ankylosing spondylitis. Recurrent anterior uveitis occurs in 30% of patients with ankylosing spondylitis and may precede or follow joint involvement. It is not correlated with disease activity. Posterior uveitis presents with floaters and impaired vision. Other systemic diseases associated with uveitis include Reiter's syndrome, Behçet's disease, sarcoidosis, inflammatory bowel disease, various infections (e.g. TB, syphilis, toxoplasmosis, toxocariasis, AIDS, herpes simplex and herpes zoster) and non-Hodgkin's lymphoma.

190. D

Bacterial conjunctivitis is usually bilateral. There may be a history of contact with a similarly infected person. In addition to giving antibiotic eye drops, avoidance of sharing face towels should be stressed.

191. A

It is important to consider the diagnosis of acute glaucoma in a patient over 50 years with a painful red eye. Urgent treatment is required to reduce the intraocular pressure and so preserve sight. This may be done medically with intravenous acetazolamide and pilocarpine should be instilled into the affected eye to constrict the pupil. Iridectomy or iridotomy may then be performed to restore normal aqueous flow. The other eye is treated prophylactically in a similar way.

192. H

The history is suggestive of herpes simplex virus associated ulcerative keratitis. Owing to inoculation from aerosols containing viral particles from patients with perioral cold sores during drilling, this is an occupational hazard for dentists. Dendritic corneal ulcers occur and are only visible with 1% fluorescein eye drops and show up green. The term keratitis refers to corneal inflammation appearing as a white spot on the cornea and represents a collection of white cells. Patients with any form of corneal ulceration should be referred urgently to hospital – delay causes loss of sight. Treatment is with aciclovir eye ointment.

193. G

Subconjunctival haemorrhage is usually harmless and involves a small-vessel bleed with blood collecting behind the conjunctiva. It resolves spontaneously but may remain bright red for a number of weeks owing to diffusion of oxygen. If recurrent then bleeding disorders and hypertension should be excluded. In head trauma a subconjunctival haemorrhage without posterior limit is associated with fractured zygomas and retrobulbar haemorrhage.

Theme: Disorders of the knee joint

194. H

A patella fracture occurs when the quadriceps contract against resistance (in this case when the foot was caught against the paving slab). Patients often hear a crack when a bone breaks. If the extensor mechanism is effectively ruptured (either by rupture of the quadriceps or patella tendons or by fracture of the patella) the patient is unable to actively extend the knee or lift the straight leg.

195. D

Osgood Schlatter's (osteochondritis of the tibial tuberosity) classically affects teenage children – particularly those who enjoy sports. A localised swelling or tender lump over the tibial tuberosity confirms the diagnosis. A tumour can not be excluded but would be very unlikely.

196. E

Primary osteoarthritis is often responsible for widespread aches and pains, whilst secondary osteoarthritis is often more specific to joints which have been damaged previously (for example following meniscectomy). Relatively minor trauma (such as playing a game of football) may lead to an acute exacerbation of symptoms and a joint effusion that understandably is uncomfortable and restricts movement.

197. B

An acutely swollen and painful knee could be a septic joint but in this case the history of heart disease and his profession make you wonder about his urate levels. (Some diuretics raise blood urate levels as can alcohol!).

Theme: Fracture complications

198. D

The deformity was probably present at the time of plaster removal but may have only just been noticed. It is too soon for a growth disturbance to become visible and at this age such a disturbance is unlikely to cause a significant (visible) deformity. Remodelling is unlikely to occur at this age.

199. G

Pain out or all proportion to what you expect the patient to be experiencing must make you think of a compartment syndrome but as the injury occurred some weeks ago this becomes very unlikely. The hand is well perfused and thus an acute ischaemic episode is unlikely. A pink or blue or sweaty hand that is very tender to touch and very stiff is likely to be a RSD.

200. B

A displaced fracture of the radius and ulna can be associated with severe swelling. If the patient has not kept his arm elevated at home and whilst in bed – the swelling could have worsened and a compartment syndrome developed. The classical features being pain out of all proportion and pain on passive stretching of the affected muscles (which could be the flexors and/or the extensors). Compartment syndrome is not usually associated with major vessel ischaemia and the hand should be pink and well perfused. An acute ischaemic event could have occurred but with this history it is much less likely.

APPENDIX 1

NORMAL RANGES

Serum	Normal Range
Albumin	36–52 g/l
Amylase	70–300 iu/l
Bicarbonate	22–28 mmol/l
Bilirubin	5–20 mmol/l
Calcium	2.20–2.60 mmol/l
Chloride	95–105 mmol/l
Creatinine kinase	23–175 iu/l
Creatinine	60–120 mmol/l
D-Dimer	< 0.3 mg/l
Gammaglutaryltransferase (GGT)	< 40 iu/l
Globulins	24–37 g/l
Immunoglobulins	
IgG	5.3–16.5 g/l
IgA	0.8–4.0 g/l
IgM	0.5–2.0 g/l
Iron	14–29 mmol/l
Iron binding capacity (TIBC)	45–75 mmol/l
Lactate dehydrogenase (LDH)	100–300 iu/l
Magnesium	0.70–1.00 mmol/l
Osmolarity	270–295 mmol/l
Phosphatase (acid)	0–4 iu/l
Phosphatase (alkaline)	40–115 iu/l
Phosphate	0.8–1.4 mmol/l
Potassium	3.5–5.0 mmol/l
Protein	62–82 g/l
Sodium	135–145 mmol/l
Thyroid function tests	
T_4	54–144 nmol/l
TSH	0.10–5.0 mU/l
T_3	0.8–2.7 nmol/l
FT_4	9–25 pmol/l
TBG	10–30 mg/l
Transaminase ALT	11–55 iu/l
Transaminase AST	13–42 iu/l
Transferrin	2–4 g/l
Urate	0.24–0.45 mmol/l
Urea	2.5–6.6 mmol/l

PLASMA

Glucose	3.0–5.9 mmol/l
Arterial blood gases [H⁺]	36–43 nmol/l
pCO₂ 4.6–6.0 kPa	
[HCO₃]	20–28 mmol/l
pO₂	10.5–13.5 kPa
Lactate	0.63–2.44 mmol/l
Pyruvate	34–80 mmol/l

CEREBROSPINAL FLUID (CSF)

Glucose	2.5–3.9 mmol/l
Protein	< 0.45 g/l
URINE	
Catecholamines	< 1.3 mmol/24 h
VMA (HMMA)	9–36 mmol/24 h
5HIAA	10–50 mmol/24 h
Microalbumin	< 30 mg/l
Creatinine clearance	60–110 ml/min

MISCELLANEOUS

Faecal fat	< 10 mmol/24 h
Xylose excretion test	
Urine excretion (25 g dose)	> 33 mmol/5 h
Urine excretion (5 g dose)	> 8 mmol/5 h
Blood xylose at 1 h (25 g dose)	2.0–4.8 mmol/l
Blood xylose at 2 h (25 g dose)	1.0–5.0 mmol/l

APPENDIX 2

USEFUL ADDRESSES

General Medical Council
178 Great Portland Street
London
W1N 6JE
Tel: 44 207 915 3481
Fax: 44 207 915 3558

First Application Service
e-mail: firstcontact@gmc-uk.org
PLAB Test Section
e-mail: plab@gmc-uk.org

British Medical Association
BMA House
Tavistock Square
London
WC1H 9JP
Tel: 44 207 387 4499

Irish Medical Association
Lower Ratmine Road
Dublin 8
Eire
Tel: 003 531 496 5588
Fax: 003 531 496 5972

PasTest Ltd
Egerton Court
Parkgate Estate
Knutsford
Cheshire
Tel: 44 (0)1565 752000
Fax: 44 (0)1565 650264
e-mail: enquiries@pastest.co.uk

NACPME
Bridgewater House
58 Whitworth Street
Manchester
M1 6BB
Tel: 44 161 957 7218
Fax: 44 161 957 7029
e-mail: nacpme@britishcouncil.org

REVISION CHECKLIST

The following themes have recently appeared in the PLAB Part 1 examination. Use this checklist in your revision.

General Medicine
- [ ] Anaemia
- [ ] Antibiotic prophylaxis
- [ ] Causes of acute breathlessness
- [ ] Causes of dysphagia
- [ ] Causes of immobility
- [ ] Causes of pneumonia
- [ ] Chest pain and its management
- [ ] Complications of anti-epileptic drugs
- [ ] Complications of diabetes
- [ ] Decision making in terminal care
- [ ] Diagnosis of acquired liver diseases
- [ ] Diagnosis of asthma
- [ ] Diagnosis of hypertension
- [ ] Diagnosis of infection
- [ ] Diagnosis of joint pain
- [ ] Diagnosis of shock
- [ ] Differential diagnosis of chest pain
- [ ] Haematological diagnosis
- [ ] Headaches
- [ ] HIV risk prevention
- [ ] Hypercalcaemia, treatment and causes
- [ ] Immediate treatment of meningitis/head injury
- [ ] Initial management of convulsions
- [ ] Investigation of chest pain
- [ ] Investigations for headaches
- [ ] Investigations relevant to urinary tract infections
- [ ] Malabsorption
- [ ] Management of arrhythmias
- [ ] Management of breast cancer
- [ ] Management of pain in terminal care
- [ ] Management of stroke/TIA
- [ ] Mechanism of poisoning
- [ ] Method of transmission of infection
- [ ] Pain relief
- [ ] Prescribing drugs in renal failure
- [ ] Prevention of jaundice and hepatitis
- [ ] Prevention and treatment of deep vein thrombosis

- ❏ Risk factors of injury in elderly
- ❏ Sudden loss of vision
- ❏ Swelling of legs
- ❏ Treatment of DVT
- ❏ Treatment of pancreatitis
- ❏ Treatment of pain relief in terminally ill patients
- ❏ Unconscious patient

Obstetrics and Gynaecology
- ❏ Antenatal screening
- ❏ Causes of incontinence
- ❏ Causes of vaginal bleeding and primary treatment
- ❏ Eclampsia and its management
- ❏ Investigations of amenorrhoea
- ❏ Investigation for ante-partum haemorrhage
- ❏ Investigations for vaginal bleeding during pregnancy
- ❏ Management of preeclampsia

Ophthalmology and ENT
- ❏ Diagnosis of earache
- ❏ Pain in the ear
- ❏ Prevention of deterioration of vision
- ❏ Sudden loss of vision
- ❏ Treatment of earache
- ❏ Treatment of red eye

Paediatrics
- ❏ Abdominal pain
- ❏ Acute vomiting in children
- ❏ Asthma
- ❏ Bleeding per vaginum
- ❏ Causes of vomiting
- ❏ Developmental delay
- ❏ Difficulty in walking
- ❏ Jaundice
- ❏ Non-accidental injuries
- ❏ Treatment of acute/chronic asthma
- ❏ Treatment of urinary tract infection

Psychiatry
- ❑ Acute confusional state
- ❑ Causes of dementia
- ❑ Differential diagnosis of confusion
- ❑ Diagnosis of depression
- ❑ Management of dementia
- ❑ Management of schizophrenia
- ❑ Psychiatric illness and its management
- ❑ Risk of suicide
- ❑ Treatment of alcoholics and drug abuse
- ❑ Treatment of psychosis

Surgery
- ❑ Antibiotic prophylaxis in surgical patients
- ❑ Complications of cholecystectomy
- ❑ Investigations of Acute abdomen
- ❑ Investigations in aortic aneurysm
- ❑ Investigations of a breast lump
- ❑ Investigations of chronic abdominal pain
- ❑ Management of burns
- ❑ Management of an ischaemic limb

INDEX

Page numbers refer to the Answers and Explanations section.

PASTEST REVISION COURSES FOR PLAB PART 1

Feeling in need of a helping hand towards success in your exams?

PasTest has over thirty years' experience in helping doctors to pass first time, with specially tailored courses to make the most of your valuable revision time.

To give you the most up-to-date information and help you to achieve the best results, we constantly update and improve our courses based on feedback from those who attend.

Our course is run by Consultants and Senior Registrars from leading London teaching hospitals, who have extensive knowledge of their specialty.

Our course material is continually updated to ensure the best possible revision for the exam. You will also receive a complete EMQ mock exam, with explanations and detailed handouts.

- **Course Content**
  Our teaching sessions are based around the PLAB Part 1 examination. The course covers core knowledge, skills and attitudes relating to all exam topics including: Accident and Emergency, Surgery, Medicine, Paediatrics, Obstetrics and Gynaecology, Trauma and Orthopaedics. Our course material includes EMQs with answers and teaching notes, an EMQ examination, tips on examination technique, detailed lecture notes for each subject and a recommended reading list.

Don't just take our word for how good our courses are ...

"Excellent revision course, complete and concise. Top quality lecturers!" Dr Geraldine Sega, Sheffield.
"The course is good, it builds a basic structure on which you can plan all your studies. It really benefitted me – I passed my exam on the first attempt." Dr Ekta Gupta, Solihull.

For queries on books and courses please call our dedicated Customer Services team on **0800 980 9814** or **+44(0)1565 752000.** Alternatively, visit our website at **www.pastest.co.uk.**